More praise for *The* ...

"Women's bodies and minds are different ...., and the best way toward a healthy, satisfying life is to embrace that difference. Provocative and thorough, *The Book of SHE* explores the mystery and alchemy of what it means to be a woman. Sara Avant Stover will guide you toward reclaiming the power and beauty of your own amazing body in this groundbreaking book."

— **Sara Gottfried, MD**, author of *The Hormone Cure*

"Sara Avant Stover knows that to give form to your dreams, you must recover your feminine field. Instead of tracking linear pathways for success, *The Book of SHE* calls for embodying your sacredness. Stover has created a priceless map for how to live from the beauty you contain."

— **Tami Lynn Kent**, author of
Wild Feminine, *Wild Creative*, and *Mothering from Your Center*

Praise for *The Way of the Happy Woman* by Sara Avant Stover

"Filled with health-promoting delight, pleasure, and truth. Just lovely."

— **Christiane Northrup, MD**, author of
Women's Bodies, Women's Wisdom

"Stover offers a wide range of practices to help readers simplify, slow down, and be in tune with natural cycles....A winner of a read."

— *Library Journal*

"*The Way of the Happy Woman* is the positive self-help product of Sara's own healing journey....Heartfelt and rich with personal stories, this book presents practical wisdom for women of all ages who are seeking to live a healthier, happier life."

— *Yoga Journal*

"In this inspiring volume, Sara Avant Stover speaks as a wise best friend, offering up secret recipes and simple ways to keep your body in sync with the four seasons.... She takes us on a personal journey of health and well-being, then sends us off as if we've completed a rite of passage, and will never be the same again."

— *Conscious Dancer*

"In *The Way of the Happy Woman*, Sara Avant Stover offers hundreds of baby steps — simple yet deceptively profound — toward living a happier, healthier, more balanced life. Even a few of these, practiced regularly, could be transformational. Highly recommended!"

— **Timothy McCall, MD**, medical editor of
Yoga Journal and author of *Yoga as Medicine*

"Rest in the nest of this beautiFULL book, and allow it to soak in and beam its wisdom to you. Your way *is* that of the happy woman, and these words will awaken, inspire, and deeply support you on your way-finding."

— **SARK**, artist, creative fountain, and author of *Glad No Matter What*

"This lovely, born-of-experience book is a primer on how to live in accord with the energies of the natural world. Clear and thoughtful, it will help you remember that even amid the demands of work, school, family, and incessant email, you're still a goddess."

— **Susan Piver**, author of *The Wisdom of a Broken Heart*
and *The Hard Questions*

THE
BOOK OF

SHE

Also by Sara Avant Stover

The Way of the Happy Woman:
Living the Best Year of Your Life

THE
BOOK OF
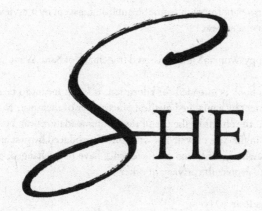
HE

YOUR HEROINE'S JOURNEY
into the HEART of
FEMININE POWER

SARA AVANT STOVER

New World Library
Novato, California

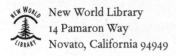

New World Library
14 Pamaron Way
Novato, California 94949

Text design by Tona Pearce Myers

Library of Congress Cataloging-in-Publication Data
Stover, Sara Avant, date.
The book of she : your heroine's journey into the heart of feminine power / Sara Avant
Stover.
    pages   cm
Includes bibliographical references and index.
ISBN 978-1-60868-289-8 (paperback) — ISBN 978-1-60868-290-4 (ebook)
1. Feminist spirituality. 2. Self-realization in women. I. Title.
BL625.7.S766 2015
204'.4082—dc23   2015022625

First printing, October 2015
ISBN 978-1-60868-289-8
Printed in Canada on 100% postconsumer-waste recycled paper

New World Library is proud to be a Gold Certified Environmentally
Responsible Publisher. Publisher certification awarded by Green Press
Initiative. www.greenpressinitiative.org

10   9   8   7   6   5   4   3   2   1

To Kogen Ananda Keith Martin-Smith, for our love.

To Sofia Diaz, for shining the light.

And

to Mary, for leading me home.

All Genders and Persuasions Welcome Here

For the sake of simplicity, the language used in this book reflects the generally accepted notion that women (biological sex) are more feminine (gender) than men and the largely masculine culture men have created. As such, it focuses on biological women who are embracing both the cultural and the spiritual aspects of the feminine. But this impulse to rediscover and embrace our Inner SHE, our inner feminine dark and light energy, is greater than biological sex. Trans women, gay men and women, and anyone longing to identify with the deeper cycles and hidden wisdom of the feminine will find this book useful. It may be harder for those who do not have the neurobiology of a woman to fully embrace these ideas, but it is by no means impossible or not recommended. Ultimately, we must embrace all of who we are, which includes all the facets of the Divine Masculine and the Divine Feminine, together as one expression of a whole, human being.

All genders and sexual orientations are fully welcomed and celebrated in this book, and to the discussions herein.

God is within her. She will not fail.

— Psalm 46:5

Contents

Part I: Preparing for the Journey

Part II: The Descent

Part III: The Initiation

Part IV: The Ascent

Part V: The Homecoming

Mary Magdalene

When a new infusion of love is needed, Mary Magdalene shows up.
Our only real choice is whether or not to cooperate.

— Cynthia Bourgeault, *The Meaning of Mary Magdalene*

Santa Fe, New Mexico; October 30, 2010

Devil's Night, some call it.

I drew the thick maroon curtains shut and opened one of the windows just a crack to let the night air in. *Click.* I switched the lamp off and pulled the covers up over my shoulders. Alone in the inn's musty guestroom.

It was the night before I was scheduled to perform the talk that I'd spent the previous four days preparing, the one I'd later give on my book tour. The next morning I'd stand, without notes or podium, before my circle of six female peers and my public speaking instructor. Just me, my story, and my heart. My body trembled, but my heart roared, "I'm ready." I could feel the fertility of something new beginning.

Shhhh. What's that?

I heard a rustling outside. And although I had never heard that sound before, I knew exactly what it was.

Nah, couldn't be.

A floor-length dress, swishing through the dark, against the cold stone patio outside. Red, I knew it to be, without even having seen it.

It sounded like a ghost or a vision coming to deliver a message, although I had never received such a message.

I rolled over to face the window. No fear, just relaxed readiness, as if waiting to begin a previously agreed-upon appointment.

I watched Her dark shadow outside the window, moving the curtains aside, lifting Her skirt carefully, and suddenly standing next to my bed. Then She climbed in bed and lay down beside me.

She smelled dusty, like She'd come from far away. And although I had never seen Her before, or even thought much of Her, I relaxed in Her presence. I only felt relief that we were together once again. At last.

She didn't introduce Herself, but I knew in the moment right before I heard Her coming who She was.

She stroked my hair, cooing to me, like I had always wished my mother had done.

"Sara, my love," she whispered, lips close to my ear, "I am here for you now, and always. You have nothing to worry about. You are my daughter. You are here to do my work in the world. Because of this, I will always take care of you. I will never be far away. I am always here with you."

We continued breathing, nose to nose, my breath warm and human, Hers ethereal and cool, like that late autumn night's breeze.

I nodded, cherishing every moment.

Yes. Yes. Thank you so much. This is right.

I rolled over, and She snuggled in behind me, wrapping Her arms around my waist. My body began to shake and sob, releasing a longing that was suddenly, unexpectedly, miraculously filled.

In our embrace, I drifted off to sleep.

And in the morning, although Mary Magdalene was physically gone, I still felt Her presence in my depths.

I felt different. Her visit planted a passion in my heart. I had no idea where it would end up leading me, but I knew that from that day on, my life would never be the same.

The Dark Side of
The Way of the Happy Woman

When there's a disappointment, I don't know if it's the end of the story.
It may just be the beginning of a great adventure.

— Pema Chödrön, *When Things Fall Apart*

Before we get started, I need to tell you a secret. In the spring of 2010, about six months before my encounter with Mary Magdalene, I experienced a perfect storm of three life-changing events that altered my path forever. Just as I signed the contract to write my first book, *The Way of the Happy Woman*, which was a lifelong dream come true, my then-boyfriend broke up with me, and my landlord asked me to move out of my idyllic home in Boulder, Colorado. Suddenly, I was bound to a six-month deadline and — despite my best attempts — I couldn't find a new home. Every possibility I came across imploded. Running out of time, and without a stable base from which to write, I received the grace of a girlfriend's invitation to move out to Ashland, Oregon, for the summer to rent a home she owned and finish the book. I packed my car, put the rest of my belongings into storage, and headed west.

Once there, I struggled to nurse my broken heart without my friends, teachers, and mentors. Instead, I dove into writing that book — something I was still not convinced I could actually pull off. Day after day, my Inner Critic pummeled me: *Why can't any of your relationships ever last? Why aren't you out enjoying the summer, like a normal person? You're such a loser. Who the hell do you think you are writing a book about happiness? You'll never be happy. What the hell is wrong with you?*

Its sneers clawed and burned inside me, until I couldn't take it anymore. One night, another familiar demon took over.

Oh no, I thought to myself. *Can this really be what I think it is? No, no. Please God, no. Not now. I've been doing so well, for so long. I am going to take some deep breaths. I am going to write in my journal. I am going to go for a walk. Call someone.*

Ha ha, nice try, Sara, it snorted, *too late.*

And the demon was right. Possessed by a dark inner force that seemed beyond my control, I got up to lock the door, draw the blinds, and head to the refrigerator to enact the perverted, ancient goddess ritual that my body knew all too well. I gathered offerings: dairy, grain, and sweets. First the ice cream. Then bowls of cereal. Bread with peanut butter. Whatever my demon wanted, she got. Until the demon said: *Enough.*

To complete the ritual, the demon dragged me into the bathroom, forced my finger down my throat, and made me vomit. Over and over and over again. Until it was all out — every last bit of it. When she was sure of that, she robotically led me to the bathroom mirror, as I wiped the carnage away from my face with the back of my wrist. There, in the mirror above the sink, *I* started to come back. I looked into my eyes — scared, sad, and hollow — like I was peering into a haunted house. I had never, *ever*, wanted to see myself like that again.

Where are you, Sara? What's happening to you? Why does this have to be so hard?

I tried to soothe my terrified reflection. *I'm so sorry, I'm so sorry, I'm so sorry; I will never do that again. I will never do that to you again.*

These pleas echoed words I had uttered to myself many times as a young woman — always in vain. I wished I could believe them this time.

The strong, willful part of me said, *Yes, it can be different.*

But my demon only cackled. *You're thirty-two fucking years old.*

Shouldn't you be free of me right now? Ha ha, nice try. You will NEVER be free of me, no matter how hard you try.

A Very Feminine Being
Having a Very Feminine Realization

A year later, I had moved back to Boulder, Colorado, found a new home, and entered into a relationship with a wonderful man named Keith, who is now my fiancé. My book had been published with much fanfare the previous spring. On the outside, it looked like the pieces of my life were coming together again, but inside I was unraveling into more and more fragments. Now I battled some new demons: searing pain in my heart, mounting anxiety, oceans of inexplicable tears, energy exploding in my pelvis and snaking up my spine, rooms spinning, my company (also called The Way of the Happy Woman®) on the brink of an unexpected bankruptcy, more visitations from Mary Magdalene, and way too many sleepless nights.

Since my root teacher in feminine spiritual practice, Sofia Diaz, was away tending to her sick mother, I resorted to seeking answers to my dilemma in the place I always had: the Patriarchy. I met with a Zen rōshi, an honored senior teacher, to help me understand what I was experiencing. During our meeting, the rōshi told me that there was nothing going on but my own neurosis, and that all I was experiencing was just a distraction from my "real" practice. He encouraged me to drop the drama and fully take my seat as imperturbable awareness. In the end, I left that encounter feeling like a broken little girl: unseen and misunderstood.

During the next few days I grew increasingly angry that the rōshi didn't "get" me and that sensitive women are too often seen as weak, crazy, and hysterical. But, most of all, I was angry with myself. A part of me believed that he was right and I wasn't strong enough to cope with the stresses of life.

A few weeks after that meeting, Sofia returned to Boulder, so I requested to meet with her privately. As I sat on a chair across from her, she instructed me to close my eyes. Then we sat up straight, deepened our breath, and arrived more fully into the moment together. The one-hour meeting I had scheduled spilled into three more hours, and I told her everything. Meeting Mary Magdalene in Santa Fe nine months earlier. The searing pain in my heart that came, mostly at night, in random episodes. The feeling that I was being completely taken over by who knows what. The bulimia relapse. The financial struggles. The rooms spinning. The tears.

Throughout our meeting, she furrowed her forehead and listened really closely, more with her eyes and her body than with her ears.

When I finally finished speaking, she cut in with a fiery rebuttal.

"First off, you need to notice your language here. Stop saying 'When *It* happens to me.' No. From now on, say, 'When *She* is communicating to me.' This is not something external to you. This *is* you. You're sovereign here, not a victim."

Then a big smile spread across her face.

"*And*, this is a Hallelujah moment!" she exclaimed, with a twinkle in her brown eyes. "When we both arrived together at the start of this session, with our eyes closed, I felt the presence of Mother Mary's blue robes in the space between us, and now I know why. I'm so happy for you, Sara!"

Then I told her about going to see the rōshi. She laughed and then pulled back, unleashing her sword once more.

"Well, what did you expect? Now, you know I love Zen. But why on earth would you even think of going to *the* most patriarchal spiritual tradition in the world to have this answered for? You are a *very* feminine being having a *very* feminine realization. That's what's going on here. So of course that rōshi couldn't help you with this. How could he? What were you thinking?"

Ouch. I let her words burn me, because I knew she was right.

"I have no idea what I was thinking," I admitted, shaking my head in disbelief.

Prior to that day, despite my extensive background in feminine spiritual practice, it had not even occurred to me to find validation for my experience within a feminine lineage. The only lineages I had ever seen acknowledged as real, bona fide paths to Awakening were masculine ones. Ultimately, those were where I had always oriented myself toward as my spiritual home.

That day things shifted one hundred and eighty degrees for me. I fully stepped off the path of practicing and Awakening like a man. I committed myself to waking up in *this* body — a woman's body — through a *feminine* spiritual practice, whatever that might entail. Sofia offered the instructions for my next steps.

"The first thing that you need to do is apologize to Mary," she ordered. "Apologize for doubting Her, for mistrusting Her, for not listening to Her, for not welcoming Her. What a huge insult to Her! She came to you to share a message and a mystical experience and you shut the door by doubting your experience and writing it off as your neuroses. First heal that. Then open up a dialogue with Her through divine communication. Ask Her to speak more loudly and clearly. Find out exactly how you two will be in dialogue. Tell Her that you are here to listen now. Tell Her that you want Her to be the center of your life."

She concluded, "This is a tremendous blessing, Sara. There's so much grace here. You're not going crazy. This is *exactly* what a feminine realization looks and feels like. This is what you've been practicing for all these years. *This is it.*"

A New Journey, a New Story

Sofia's reframing of my experience helped me to understand that my collapse was really my gateway to what has been the hardest, most rewarding, and most miraculous journey of my life so far — my Heroine's Journey.

The process of writing *The Way of the Happy Woman* awakened old and deeply wounded parts of myself that I thought I had healed through the very process I was teaching. All of the therapy, yoga, meditation, and healing work that I had done over the prior decade felt like it had flown out the window. None of it worked when bulimia, which I had begun to experience when I was sixteen, began resurfacing, seemingly out of the blue.

I responded by trying to hide in the familiar, safe harbor of my shameful silence and secrecy. *Make sure everyone thinks things are "good" and "perfect." Don't show your true feelings. Keep the family secrets safe.* I didn't know any other way to be. I felt that there were some things about myself that were just *too* shameful to speak of — to anyone.

My meeting with Sofia also revealed that when my carefully controlled "Citadel of Sara" started to crumble, I tried to guide my inner life with the same deranged masculine drive that had served as the shaky foundation of my entire existence. I tapped into the same compulsive, restless, trying-to-prove-my-worth energy — only this time I did it with a much subtler, more "spiritual" outlet. The reality was that I still pushed myself in damaging ways — even though I taught others not to. I still tried to control my body and my surroundings. I still mistrusted my instincts and inner guidance. And the most dangerous part of it all was that *I* was responsible for this abuse — not my parents, the media, my teachers, my report card, or the bathroom scale. It was me. *I* was the one who was continually tightening the strings of my invisible corset, making it harder and harder to breathe, feel, or move, much less flower.

When I took a closer look, I realized this wasn't just *my* problem. It's also *yours*, for it's a collective wound that we're all suffering. We're all sick with the same disease — to the point where it's so commonplace that we think it's normal. Specifically, we've gotten so consumed with being outwardly successful that we have no idea what it means to have a successful *inner life*. In little or large ways, we're all disconnected from our centers, betraying our deepest selves — our SHEs — in some fashion.

This has become the way of the world. The soul, especially the elusive, *feminine* soul, is nearly extinct. We live only on the material plane, completely cut off from our real roots in the spiritual plane, and this causes a grave and painful separation from the sustenance in our depths. So here we all are, running faster than we can — or even should — to flee this pain. No wonder we're all exhausted.

Like me, you've probably reached a certain place in your life where nothing really fits anymore, and you feel that something is sorely missing. What once felt good now feels bad, and this change has made you disoriented. You're at a crossroads. A crisis in your womanhood. And if you aren't in that place now, it's very likely that you will be soon. But don't despair. These crisis points are necessary evolutionary pivots for us as women. They initiate times when we're called to detach from our smaller sense of self to graduate into living the fuller spectrum of our womanhood, humanity, and divinity.

We're all living at the tail end of a long, patriarchal dominion, where more is always more. Reason rules above all else. Black and white. Good and bad. However, by living in this way, we are all still walking around as little girls in women's bodies. According to the old way of thinking, we're supposed to live in a very linear way: get our periods, get married, have a baby, live happily ever after. Yet when we force ourselves into these ideals, we are inevitably disappointed.

In reality, our lives as women cannot be represented by a straight line. Rather, our journeys take us through a series of circular initiations. Each crisis that lowers us into the dark underworld calls us to listen to and trust ourselves in ever-deepening ways. We have been led to believe that partnering with our darkness will make us crazy, but the truth is that only denying our darkness can do that.

There's tremendous power locked inside our darkness, for darkness is one half of creation, the gateway to our holy power. Only through our own direct experience of standing unarmored in the extremes can we realize that SHE knows no difference between good and bad, pain and pleasure, ugly and beautiful. Only then can our greatest wounds become the portal for Her to fill and bless all the cells in our bodies and all the corners of our lives with unconditional love.

It's time to wake up to the truth that we are our own worst enemies, and that the invisible corsets we have been wearing are slowly killing our passions, instincts, and connections to life itself. Tied up so tightly through the constrictions of our own Inner Patriarchs, we don't know what it is to inhale the feminine all the way in and down. We have not yet been initiated into the feminine — a realm that celebrates uncertainty and complexity, rather than rigid either-or convictions. Without this, we don't truly know what *being* a woman *feels* — much less *looks* — like. We live in a time when a woman's true genius is still deeply feared and misunderstood, and despite the increased awareness of so many things concerning women, we're still going to need a lot of support in unearthing and understanding our real, feminine gifts.

To understand these gifts, we need to realize that our limitations hold our greatest strengths. We can be struggling and evolving simultaneously. Just as the Buddha taught, within suffering is the cessation of suffering.

Sofia was right. When my bulimia resurfaced, it actually showed me that my practice really *was* working, for it had made me strong enough to look my deepest fears in the eye. When I finally did, it wasn't the pretty process that typically graces the cover of yoga magazines, but it did allow me to experience union — the real goal of yoga — by healing at the *root* level.

Throughout my entire journey to becoming a more whole, empowered woman, which I spell out in this book, I knew that I was transforming my inner hell into a collective heaven in order to help other women do the same. Even as masculine frames of reference labeled my pain and confusion as *mess, failure,* and *neuroticism,* my hope of serving other sisters fueled me through my darkest moments. I wanted my demons not only to liberate me, but also to help liberate *you.*

We need a model for true, feminine empowerment now, because the world is changing quickly. We desperately need a coherent road map to inwardly navigate these massive shifts. In less than a decade, the scales have tipped, and more and more women are rising into power in the West. Recent studies reveal that "the majority of working wives will out-earn their husbands in the next generation," and in most urban U.S. areas, "single women with no children in their 20s outearned their male peers."[1] Similarly, an article in *The Atlantic*, titled "The End of Men," revealed that "women dominate today's colleges and professional schools — for every two men who will receive a BA this year, three women will do the same. Of the 15 job categories projected to grow the most in the next decade in the U.S., all but two are occupied primarily by women."[2]

These advances can be dangerous if we don't understand what it looks like to truly triumph through our distinctly feminine rites of passage. We'll live in shame and secrecy if we don't bring into the light the very initiatory transitions that could deliver us the power that is our birthright. Along the same lines, if we keep in shadow the feminine strengths that arise out of our vulnerability, we will remain confused about our power and erroneously look for it in the wrong places.

We can't be powerful like men are because we're *not* men. Feminine empowerment is always right under our noses, yet it continues to elude us because we think it's a flaw rather than a strength. In fact, it's so obvious and natural that we keep missing it.

My sincerest hope is that you will find in these pages the architecture of your own initiation into empowerment. You will be able to place what you think are your neuroses, weaknesses, addictions, or need-to-be-fixed parts of yourself into a favorable, even devotional, light. You will discover the tools and perspectives necessary to turn your inner demons into the very freedom, creativity, joy, and power that you currently seek by trying to *deny* them. You will learn that your poison *is* your medicine, that *you* are the only medicine woman who can perform that alchemy, and that this sacred play must unfold within the crucible of your own imperfectly perfect *female* body.

Who Is SHE?

Some call her Sophia. Others call her Kuan Yin, Mary, Pachamama, Buffalo Woman, Grandmother Spider, Isis, Shakti, the Mother.

She's the sparkle in your eyes, the wind weaving through trees, the leap of your dog through the hills outside.

She's the very breath you're breathing right now. The roll of thunder outside. The pulsation in your body that you've grown numb to. The blood in your underwear, the bloat in your belly.

We all have to find Her, and in finding Her, we must learn how and what to call Her.

I call her SHE.

SHE's the one who won't let you hide anymore. Who lives inside you, even when you ignore Her.
SHE's the one who draws in anything and everything that's both good and deplorable about your life. SHE's your expansion and your contraction, your love and your hate.
SHE's everywhere because SHE's everything.
And yet, SHE's so subtle that you could miss Her. Most of us do.

SHE seems unpredictable, but there's great wisdom to Her grace. SHE's a trickster, with a wicked sense of humor.

SHE's here to remind you: you're destined for more than just suffering your suffering.

SHE won't let you fall asleep to the song of your soul.

SHE doesn't care if you're uncomfortable, SHE only cares that you wake up to the truth of who you are.

Most every woman has forgotten Her, and yet, SHE's alive and well.

Even if you think you've never met Her, SHE's always been with you. SHE will never leave you. No matter what.

SHE can't be controlled. SHE can't be acquiesced into becoming anything other than SHE.

SHE's an unconventional compass by which to navigate life.

SHE's a genius, here to lead you home to yours.

And SHE will enter in any way that SHE can.

Your Embodied Heroine's Journey:
The Portal to Your Power

Even within the feminist movement, we ignore the power and splendor of the female body. We keep looking outside of us for the answers to our struggles when the only place to find them is within. We talk about the Sacred Feminine, the goddess Kali, the phoenix rising from the ashes — and yet we deny and ignore these very embodied processes within our own bodies. We *are* the creators *and* the destroyers. We hold within us the power to give birth to divinity, in ourselves, and in all things. We *are* the miracle we've been praying for. Pulsing within the cells and soul of every woman resides this ancient remembrance, waiting to be stirred. As women, we are simultaneously the sacred matter of life *and* the power to transform it. When we root ourselves in this power, *Her* power, we discover that the very blueprint for the empowerment we've been seeking in our accomplishments is already scripted in our own DNA.

This journey will transpire in your body, *not* in your head. The feminine journey is relational, cyclical, and alchemical — *not* linear and logical. If we continue to view our cyclical crises as failures, we will always feel like we're missing the mark. We will continue to feel the longing to unite with the Sacred Feminine within us, but we will never arrive there. SHE will stay in our heads, in people and images and pursuits outside of us, never entering our hearts, wombs, and cells. Why would you even try to realize the Divine Feminine anywhere else but *in the cycles of creation and destruction that live in your own body*? You will never find Her anywhere else.

Your body and your cycles are your greatest blessing as a woman. They hold the keys to your Heroine's Journey, allowing you to know and live your true power, in very practical ways, every day. Your body is the chalice within which the miracle of creation occurs.

Your challenges hold the only energy that can cure your exhaustion and annihilate your depression. Like a mother whose jaw drops in rapture when she draws her babe to her breast for the first time, you must allow the creativity that is part yours and part beyond you — and the divine love that emerges from it — to heal you, all the way to the core. Remember that creation isn't predictable; it's dark, muddy, mysterious, and painful. Art isn't *out there*, it's *in here*. Infinite creativity is your natural state. The magic that pours forth from the integration of your dark and light sides is *always* only euphoric, beatific, and an expression of divine perfection itself.

About This Book

This book is the hard-earned creative miracle that has arisen from the ashes of my own Heroine's Journey. The insights that I share here are due to Her grace. This book is Her transmission, through me, into you. At this book's heart lives my utmost conviction that women who do their inner work *can* and *will* change the world. Above all, this book is an initiation into love. Real, deep, everlasting love.

I've compiled here the best — and worst — of my own psychological, spiritual, and embodied studies over the past twenty years. In these pages is the fruition of my self-understanding, research, insights, and wisdom gleaned from my ongoing daily practice, retreats, intimate relationships, and beloved teachers, mentors, and therapists; and the in-the-trenches work I've been doing with thousands of women, of all ages and ethnicities, around the world for the past thirteen years. Over the past four of these, I've exclusively taught pieces of the journey that I'll recount for you in this book, through my virtual and in-person programs: the SHE School (the group mentoring and women's spiritual practice community that was formerly called the Red Tent; www.TheSHESchool.com); Reversing Our "Curse" (www.ReversingOurCurse.com); and the annual SHE Retreat (www.SHEretreat.com).

Since some aspects of this journey must be experienced instead of taught, and the feminine teaches most potently through storytelling, I have woven my own narrative throughout these pages to reveal some of the deeper, subtler insights that can arise when you fully commit to Her path.

As you read these pages and embark on your own journey, I hope you will share your personal story with others. Currently, this world is starved for stories of women on the spiritual path. Without these, we don't have a way to validate or make sense of our experiences, and our deeper truths remain hidden in silence and confusion. As women, we need to tell our stories of how we experience the divine and not feel wrong or crazy for doing so.

The work I share in this book fuses ancient practices from two-thousand-year-old wisdom traditions with the latest scientific research and discoveries in order to address the complex problems of our contemporary lives through one simple, elegant model. It turns our current paradigm for success and empowerment on its head, teaching us that everything in our outer world is based on the unseen, inner one. By changing the inner, we change the outer — *not* the other way around. Through relinquishing our chronic busyness, we open up the space to increase our capacity to be present and truly enjoy this precious life.

As part of the process to mature and Awaken, we must confront the unhealed pain of our pasts. At the same time, instead of always trying to fix what's wrong with us, we need to simply learn how to love ourselves. This book rewrites our journey into power as modern women by reviving a revamped archetype of "the Heroine" that is most needed in order for us to best face our most pressing current dilemmas.

This template of a woman's path to complete empowerment — in all dimensions — as the Heroine's Journey offers us the means to live from our hearts. It reminds us that we find true success only by continually turning our conventional minds toward the contemplation of deeper truths, while being fully present to all the moments of our own lives. This journey grounds us in the holiness of our female bodies and teaches us that it's exactly through our failures that real, liberated womanhood can be born.

My own perceived failure — from bulimia to near-bankruptcy, to the collapse of my self-identity — opened the door to this book, prompting me to update and build upon the wisdom from my previous book to provide a broader, deeper, and more nuanced perspective of a modern woman's initiation into her true *feminine* power. While *The Way of the Happy Woman* focused more on the external aspects of our womanhood through seasonal lifestyle rituals, yoga, meditation, and nutrition, this book looks more closely at our internal ones — our psyches and souls. To fully flower, we need to use *both* external and internal approaches, together.

How to Use This Book

The first step in any initiation is activating radical trust. Trust that you are here for a reason, even if that reason is not yet clear to you. Life doesn't happen *to* you, it happens *for* you. You don't need to know what, exactly, you're looking for, or what you want from this journey. You just have to acknowledge that a deeper part of you was called here. Own your place on this path and walk it, with me and many others, with dignity. This book is one of the many ways that SHE is calling you. Whether you're eighty or twenty, or any age in between, welcome.

This is *your* journey. Nothing is too taboo, too wonderful, too shameful, too grotesque, or too brilliant to lay down here. Bring all of yourself.

No part of you will be rejected or turned away. Throughout, remember that *you* are your own best teacher. Use your experience reading this book to become a connoisseur of your deepest Self.

Some Things for You to Know before Diving In

- This is a self-help book that's also *not* a self-help book. This isn't a paint-by-numbers model that you can simply check things off of and "do." It's more like a scavenger hunt. I drop the bread crumbs, but you need to string them together within your lived experience.
- This book operates on four different levels: my personal journey, your journey and teachings for how you can partake in it, your own experience, and our collective sisterhood experience as we take this journey together.
- Some of my teachings are prescriptive, giving you exact steps to follow. Others are more demonstrative, pointing to a deeper, more organic current of how transformation could transpire.
- It's important to appreciate all the little celebrations along the way.
- You can't fail or do this journey "wrong," nor can you do it perfectly.
- This isn't a religious book. It's a very personal, direct, lived experience of the divine that's available to all of us in everyday life — regardless of any specific faith.
- You can start exactly where you are. Trust your process. Let yourself be where you are.
- We're all in different stages of the Heroine's Journey. Don't compare yourself to anyone else.
- With that in mind, this book is designed to be followed in order. It's a methodical, steady progression. *Do not jump ahead*. You need to engage in every part sequentially to experience the fruits. Don't exclude or gloss over anything — especially the parts that you have resistance to. As you read, do all the practices accompanying each chapter. This is both a book to read *and* a process to *live*.

- A steady — ideally, daily — spiritual practice needs to accompany this book in order for this journey to fully take hold. I recommend a practice that includes conscious embodiment (yoga, tai chi, chi gung, etc.), concentration and compassionate awareness (meditation), self-inquiry, and devotion (prayer). My approach to all of these elements is outlined in *The Way of the Happy Woman*, so in this book I simply expand upon rather than reiterate that material. If you're already well established in your own daily practice, feel free to continue on with that.

- This is meant to be a three-dimensional process. Don't be a lone Heroine. The Buddha taught the importance of the triple gem: the Buddha (one's own Awakened essence), the Sangha (one's spiritual family and community), and the Dharma (the teachings). Employ all three of these as you read this book. (Readers who don't have a spiritual community can experience this journey with our free, virtual sisterhood, which I will discuss at the end of this section.) If you work with this book in this way, you will experience significant transformation in your life.

- I mention my teacher Sofia a lot. I hold this teacher-student relationship as one of my most treasured assets. Without her guidance I would never have embarked on this journey, and this book wouldn't exist. I stand firm that, in order to evolve, we need to root ourselves in living wisdom lineages and work closely with teachers, rather than adhering to the now commonplace false belief that we can do it all ourselves. Unless we work within lineages, the profound wisdom of the ancients that is needed to move our world forward will die. This doesn't mean, however, that we put our teachers on pedestals. Rather, we can regard them as our spiritual friends, a few steps ahead of us on the journey.

- I often refer to the larger SHE as Mary, for that is primarily how I experience Her. Please insert your own experience of SHE wherever necessary if this interpretation doesn't work for you.

- This work lasts a lifetime *and* transformation can happen in an instant. Relinquish any expectations for what your journey will look like or how it will end. Practice patience — the word the Buddha is said to have used the most in his teachings!

• The more you put into this, the more you'll get out of it.

Hold off on making drastic changes in your life while you're on this journey. Wait until you've completed the whole thing and then let the dust settle. Over time, the answers for your next steps will appear. Don't force things to happen before they're ready to.

Finally, be patient and gentle with yourself as you follow these three stages of learning:

1. Observe and become aware of how the new concepts operate within and around you.
2. Gradually layer the practices and perspectives into your daily life.
3. Master the practices to the point where you're able to consistently use what you've learned and the practices have become second nature.

After you've practiced everything offered here to your fullest capacity, take what works for you, revisit it as often as needed, and feel free to let go of any parts that don't resonate with you.

Note: During this process, a free "SHE Circle" is available to you online. It's a safe holding environment for women who are embarking on this journey or have already started to follow the path. In this circle, you can ask for support and share your celebrations, challenges, and insights as you journey through this book and beyond. To join our sisterhood, please visit www.TheBookofSHE.com/practices.

How This Book Is Organized

While everything that I share has come out of my own direct, lived experience, I acknowledge that I am standing on the shoulders of giants. The wisdom accrued here comes from many sources — both living and dead, seen and unseen. After two decades of deep inner work, I have pieced together the very best of those who have most served me along the way.

The whole arc of the journey came together for me in a revelation from Mary during one of my solitary retreats. In a few moments, SHE imprinted this entire book into my heart, and it was then up to me to spend the next two and a half years putting words to it. Through this precise configuration, I have been able to weave fragments of wisdom that were once disparate into a pilgrimage to feminine empowerment — and ultimately into your own self-realization and emergence as an integrated human being.

Together we'll embark on this Heroine's Journey in five parts.

In part I, we prepare for our pilgrimage. We get clear on what, exactly, the Heroine's Journey *is*. We renounce our "normal" lives, explore the wounding that brought us here, and learn how to become loving mothers to ourselves. We build a strong, safe, and compassionate container to hold our process, while getting clear on the essential pieces of creating an enduring, effective feminine spiritual practice and living a SHE-centered life. We craft our intentions for the journey and directly meet our own Inner SHEs to guide us.

From this firm foundation, we descend into the underworld in part II. We learn how to partner with the power of darkness by facing the Dark Goddess and our inner demons head-on. We dialogue with our Inner Critic and other inner saboteurs. We meet our "shadow sides," our addictions, and our neuroses. We shed our perfectionist standards and surrender to the inevitable messes of our lives. To conclude our time in the underworld, we learn how to cocreate with our divine natures through the embodied cycles of the Heroine's Journey that hold the key to our feminine power yet are cloaked in our shame: our PMS, menses, perimenopause, and menopause. We practice dying during the still-point of each month so that we can face our final exhales without any regrets. Calling on the wisdom of our own Inner Crones, we learn to speak and live our truth, regardless of external opinions or agendas.

The bonfire of our initiation transpires in part III. Here, we meet the "fairy godmother" of our transformation. We learn the feminine art of feeding, rather than warring with, our inner demons, and we rewire the crucial, erotic connection between our wombs and our hearts. Through participating with the fertile darkness in the crucible of our sacred hearts, we tremble at our edges and surrender to SHE who is greater than us. In doing so, we're transfigured by the light — and reborn.

In part IV, we ascend. From the burial ground of the heart, we heal our relationship with the Divine Masculine, discover our Virgin sovereignty, and rekindle our capacities to create magic. Through this, we dip into the holy river of the Tao, embrace our nobility by reconnecting with our Magical Little Girls within, and unlock valuable inner resources — the qualities of the Awakened heart and mind. Through this, we remember that creativity heals us, and we enjoy a rush of new energy when we unlock the genius once hidden in our demons.

We now have all we need for our homecoming in part V. Full with the fruits of our inner journey, we return to the place from which we started, ready to bless the world with our innate gifts. From this holy wholeness, we sing the songs of our SHEs for the world.

Start Now

More than ever before, the world desperately needs the balance and the reclamation of the right use of power by both the Divine Feminine *and* the Divine Masculine. It needs your help to regain its spiritual center and to flower once more. So please, don't wait to start your journey. You're part of the solution. Choose to open, create, and evolve. Become a female role model who's conscious, comfortable in her own skin, and Awake. Unleash your distinctly feminine power and see this world not through the eyes of competition and fear, but through the eyes of love.

Stand firm in the knowledge that the world *is* ready for this. The Divine Mother is the goddess most loved and revered by millions around the world — across all genders, ethnicities, and religions. SHE's right here, alive and well; we've just forgotten how to see Her. Yet even when hidden from view, SHE binds us all together in our suffering and our faith. Within our love for Her lies our love for ourselves and all that is innocent in the world. There rests our salvation and the truth that we can still turn this world around, together.

Come now, take my hand. Let's begin, for life is precious and passes all too quickly. Your Heroine's Journey awaits.

Part I

Preparing for the Journey

This is my life, not a fairy tale....I have to go to the woods, and I have to meet the wolf, or else my life will never begin.

— Dr. Clarissa Pinkola Estés, *Women Who Run with the Wolves*

Mother Mary

Darien, Connecticut; January 1985

The *tick, tick, tick* of the red plastic Hello Kitty alarm clock on my bedside table reminds me that it's past my bedtime. Burt rests on his blue blanket at my feet. I hear his rolling purrs as he presses his orange paws, one after the other, into its plump threads.

My parents' shoes *click clack* on the wood floor of the hallway outside my room. I sit up, reach for Burt, and pull him up into my arms. I lie back down, roll to my right, and curl my knees up toward him, now at my chest. Next to Hello Kitty, Mother Mary, a First Communion gift from my godmother, sits inside Her petite brass frame.

She gazes placidly down at Her delicate hands, which rest in Her lap, one on top of the other. I want to be there too, protected by Her crown of five golden stars. I want Her to cradle me in the folds of that dusty rose dress. To feel that safe, calm, peaceful, and pure.

Mommy and Papa's voices thunder.

Is the wall shaking now, or is that just me? My stomach hurts. I squeeze Burt more tightly, and he rubs his wet nose against my chin. I wonder if my sisters are asleep or if they too are awake and afraid. I fix my eyes on Mary. I don't know what else to do.

I whisper to Her:

Our Father, who art in heaven,
Hallowed be Thy name.
I hear more yelling.

Tears drench my face. My body heaves to hide the sound that wants to spill from it. I keep my eyes locked on Mary.

Thy kingdom come,
Thy will be done,
on earth as it is in heaven.

White light pours into the knot in my tummy. Am I awake or dreaming? The pain there starts to soften. I long for the morning, when my room is bright and my alarm rings and it's oatmeal for breakfast and sitting in the back of the school bus, laughing with Carolyn.

I don't hear anything.

Give us this day our daily bread,
and forgive us our trespasses,
as we forgive those who trespass against us;

My eyelids are heavy. Mary fades into the darkness along with the rest of my room. My body relaxes and becomes still. Burt is asleep.

and lead us not into temptation,
but deliver us from evil.
For thine is the kingdom,
and the power, and the glory,
for ever and ever.
Amen.

Chapter 1

Leaving Your "Normal" Life

If you are always trying to be normal,
you will never know how amazing you can be.

— Maya Angelou, *Rainbow in the Cloud*

I'm going to tell you a story you've never heard before. I'm going to tell you a fairy tale the way it's meant to be told. It's not a story where, in a land far, far away, an evil witch torments you until Prince Charming saves you. It's one that transpires in your own body. One where you perpetually plague *yourself*, until you wake up to the realization that you're the only one who can liberate *yourself* through your own true love. In this story, you embrace the best and *worst* parts of yourself, and in so doing, you transform your obstacles into opportunities to become the woman you know you're born to be.

We come to know our true potential through opening to whatever life offers us — the good, the bad, *and* the ugly. The mess *is* the portal to our womanhood. Our bodies know this well. The greatest initiations of our lives, birth and death, are painful, grotesque even — no matter how hard we try to make them otherwise. Who are we to think that everything that transpires between those two milestones should be hunky-dory?

The Chinese character for *crisis* includes those for both *danger* and *opportunity*. We need to acknowledge the truth about our naturally tumultuous womanhood, and, together, weave a larger, more inclusive narrative of empowerment that acknowledges that chaos and destruction are *always* half of our reality. Birth and death, joy and sorrow, gain and loss, success and failure — these are all partners. You can never have one without the other. It's exhausting to try to get more of the good by pushing away all the bad. Clinging and craving create a game we can *never* win.

Instead of freezing, fighting, or yearning to be rescued, how can we learn to flow through these natural fluctuations? How can we reunite our smart minds with our even wiser hearts and bodies, so we're not living in a constant state of inner war? How can we learn to trust that disasters are often thresholds to the very miracles we seek? Becoming a Heroine is a choice. It involves being willing to view our lives through a new, more honest and accurate lens. It beckons us to unlearn everything we've ever been taught about what it looks like to be a successful, happy, and powerful woman.

As a devoted spiritual practitioner and closet psychology nerd for two decades and counting, I've noticed two things. First, those practitioners immersed in the spiritual world need to embrace a better understanding of their own psyches. Without psychological health, spiritual practitioners get lost in the weeds of spiritual bypassing, a phrase coined by one of my teachers, John Welwood, in 1984.[1] They seek only to transcend the mess of life and embrace the light, blissful side of reality.

Second, those experts in the psychology field need to expand their view into a larger, spiritual context. If we don't incorporate spirituality, we get stuck analyzing and rehashing old childhood wounds without ever meeting the part of ourselves that never has, and can never be, broken.

Currently, neither approach is whole, and the consequences are grave. As we move forward, we need to understand that cultivating psychological health isn't the end of the road; it's the launching point of the spiritual journey. We need both, in different degrees at different stages of our lives, in order to weather the inner work required to become fully functioning adults *and* fully realizing spiritual beings.

Welcome to Your Heroine's Journey

This Heroine's Journey merges the spheres of psychology and spirituality into a singular, embodied psycho-spiritual path to psychological wholeness, empowerment, and, ultimately, full spiritual realization. It is *not* the same as Joseph Campbell's "Hero's Journey," a singular, central narrative of becoming that is found woven throughout diverse religions, regions, and times (e.g., the stories of Moses, Odysseus, Christ, Gautama the Buddha, and more modern, pop-culture adventures such as *Star Wars, Indiana Jones, The Matrix,* and *The Wizard of Oz*).

The Hero's Journey follows the distinct phases of Departure / Separation, Initiation, and Return and was conceived by Campbell in 1949 with only men in mind. Women, who were primarily housewives at the time, were believed to not need to undergo the journey.[2] The Heroine's Journey, therefore, takes into account a woman's neurobiology as well as her separate cultural history. The goal of the Hero's Journey is individuation. The goal of the Heroine's Journey includes individuation but then transcends it to also include spiritual liberation.

The more gender-specific map of the Heroine's Journey better helps us to understand the unique twists and turns that our initiation into empowered womanhood entails. It ensures that we arrive at our desired destination — living in full alignment with our deepest, truest feminine nature. This map has primarily been hidden from us as women, thus contributing to our sense of disconnection from and confusion about our feminine strengths. When women everywhere have a detailed map to look to, we are less likely to think that we're lost or derailed when embroiled in a struggle. With a unifying perspective about our pathway into empowered womanhood, suddenly what we have previously labeled as "strange," "shameful," and "neurotic" becomes normal, natural, and even necessary for our growth. Elements we once saw as scary and dangerous become the void we all must leap into in order to taste our full potential.

With such a map we discover that the way out doesn't come from targeting and eradicating what's wrong with us. Instead, we learn to recognize that we simply need to be kind and loving to ourselves, no matter what. Even in our darkest moments, we're not off track at all. We're actually exactly where we need to be. When we cultivate embodied wholeness *and* ultimate freedom through the practices described in this book, we, as goddesses incarnate, can perfume the world with the fragrant balm of love, compassion, and sweetness that it needs now more than ever.

In order for the Heroine's Journey to take root, it must expand to encompass the two levels of reality that we're always operating within — the relative and the Absolute. *Relative reality* is the world of duality. Night and day. Life and death. Light and dark. Good and bad. Pain and pleasure. Male and female. It lives within time and space, and our perception of it is housed within "I," "me," and "mine" (our egos, or our conditioned personalities). *Absolute reality* is transcendent. It exists in the ever-arising now-ness — beyond time and space, duality, and our perceived sense of separateness. It lives within us all along; yet, as all spiritual traditions teach, we often live in delusion, forgetting our true nature of open, loving, limitless, spacious interconnectedness. Of course, the relative can only operate within the Absolute — only one can be real.

When we extend the Heroine's Journey to address these two dimensions, it does not leave out *any* part of us — human or divine. It shows us that once we become whole and individuated, we can't stop there. We must go to the furthest reaches of our human potential. We must extend our hearts and minds, beyond our hurts, closures, and limiting beliefs, to express divine love and wisdom right here, in this world, and in this most ordinary of moments.

Also, because of our intimate relationship as women with nature, the Heroine's Journey happens simultaneously in the world *and* in our physical bodies, but it *always* begins within. We then need a more detailed guide for how to work with our female bodies — particularly our cycles, the cornerstone of our womanhood, which conversations about feminine empowerment still bafflingly ignore.

The Key Ingredients of the Heroine's Journey

- **Journaling** to cleanse our minds of debris, metabolize emotions, and connect to our inner wisdom by writing down our free-flowing, unedited stream of consciousness.
- **Buddhist meditation** to help us become the observers of our

experiences by cultivating "witness consciousness," and to activate our resilience by "being with what is" within an inner mood of loving-kindness.

- **Divine Feminine practices** to awaken our inner goddess natures through play, dance, sacred sexuality, pleasure, communing with like-minded soul sisters, and spending time in nature.

- **Devotional practices** to open our hearts and invoke a disposition of surrender through prayer and living our lives as offerings.

- **Archetypes** to help access latent parts of our psyches that are needed to unlock more of our divine potential in a new season of life.

- **SHE Cycles** to heal shame about the core of our womanhood, train ourselves in partnering with mini-cycles of death and rebirth within our monthly hormonal cycles, and taproot the infinite creative power of the Goddess that lives within every woman.

- **Explorations of childhood trauma** through practices like connecting to the earth — inner and outer — and activating Mother *and* Father Love in order to feel safe and at home in the world, even amid tremendous instability and uncertainty.

- **Shadow work** to reroute lifelong patterns of self-sabotage into pathways for empowered sovereignty.

- **Voice Dialogue**, a method developed by psychologists Hal and Sidra Stone in the 1970s, to allow us to map out and speak with all of our inner "selves," discovering what each needs and has to offer. It opens the doorway to greater self-understanding and acceptance to "end the war within" between our disowned and dominant inner selves by consciously communicating and collaborating with them.

The final two essentials — **SHE Yoga**, which includes women's yin and flow yoga as well as yogic breathing and energy cultivation practices to enliven and awaken our physical and subtle bodies, and **seasonal living** to align our entire life with nature's cycles while eating responsibly grown, seasonal, local food suited for our individual constitutions — can be found in *The Way of the Happy Woman*.[3]

As we explored in the Introduction, more women are stepping into power today than at any other time in history, and it is clear that we all need a new model to follow. In 1990, Maureen Murdock wrote a groundbreaking book called *The Heroine's Journey*.[4] A Jungian therapist, Murdock worked with women between the ages of thirty and fifty and noticed a commonality: they (as well as their male counterparts) all disconnected from their feminine essence to "get to the top." These observations compelled her to adapt Joseph Campbell's Hero's Journey for women, and in so doing, she discovered a *different* recurring pattern, or monomyth of individuation, which existed throughout the lives of all the women with whom she was working. My work expands upon hers and reflects the stages I experienced within my own life and witnessed within the lives of the women I mentor — spanning from psychology to spirituality, victimhood to empowerment, relative to Absolute.

Like the Hero's Journey, the Heroine's Journey moves clockwise along a circular path. In both instances, we end up exactly where we started, but with a radically different view. At the end of our lives, we can see the entire arc of our existence as one large cycle, and we can also see lots of mini-cycles throughout our lives. In fact, we can be at several stages of the journey at the same time. Here is an overview of the main stages.

The Thirteen Stages of the Heroine's Journey

Feminine time has long been kept by the moon, which passes through thirteen cycles every year. Our journey also moves through thirteen separate — yet interconnected — cycles.

Part I: *Preparing for the Journey*

1. Leaving Your "Normal" Life: After living as a Father's Daughter, aligning with patriarchal definitions of success and becoming pseudo-male in order to survive your family of origin, you discover worldly success (e.g., money, fame, status) by repudiating your femininity as weak, manipulative, or crazy. Then, burned out and disenchanted with outer success

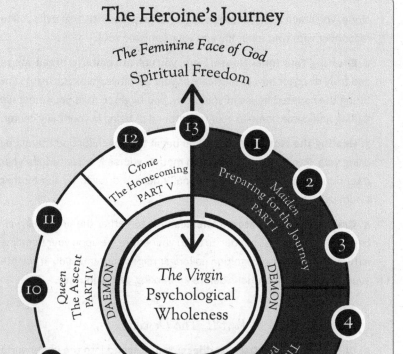

The Heroine's Journey

The Feminine Face of God
Spiritual Freedom

1. Leaving Your "Normal" Life
2. Entering Your Inner House
3. Healing the Mother Wound
4. Crafting a SHE-Centered Life
5. Dancing with the Dark Goddess
6. Ending the War Within
7. Unlocking the Magic in Your SHE Cycles
8. Meditating on Your Mortality
9. Unveiling the Sacred Heart of *Real* Feminine Power
10. Turning On Your Brights
11. Marrying the Divine Masculine
12. Birthing Your Beautiful Life
13. Becoming a Whole and Holy Heroine

alone, you reach a major crossroads or suffer a life crisis that calls you to reconnect with your inner life and your feminine soul.

2. Entering Your Inner House: Here, you unlearn patterns of self-abuse and truly discover how to take care of your sensitive, feminine being. Entering the haunted house of your body, you begin to melt your Inner Ice Ceiling and come home to your real ground of being in your belly center.

3. Healing the Mother Wound: You begin to heal childhood trauma by using your own loving awareness to mother yourself, while turning your attention toward being unconditionally held and loved by the Mother Goddess.

4. Crafting a SHE-Centered Life: It's time to gather the practices, values, and perspectives needed to build your entire life upon your feminine nature. Since outer recognition no longer reigns supreme, you articulate your deepest life intentions before embarking on the journey.

Part II: The Descent

5. Dancing with the Dark Goddess: You descend into the underworld and adjust your eyes to discern between the "two types of darkness." You meet the Dark Goddess, your demons, and your shadow behavior, while ventilating your secrets and owning your projections.

6. Ending the War Within: Unmasking your demons to discover the true faces of your inner saboteurs, you meet your greatest allies. You start to take back the power in your dark side.

7. Unlocking the Magic in Your SHE Cycles: Here, you discover how to create your new, SHE-centered life from your own sacred anatomy. You participate in the mini–Heroine's Journey of death and rebirth that happens through your monthly lunar and hormonal cycles, and you use these cycles as trainings in how to gracefully weather life's challenges.

8. Meditating on Your Mortality: Prepare for your greatest rite of passage of all — your death, and the deaths of those you love most — through dying each month on the new moon and the first day of your cycle. Live a life without regret through respecting the wisdom in your perimenopause and menopause. Activate your Inner Crone to help you shed old agendas and identifications, completely "see" and trust the darkness of your inner world above all else, and create the life that's right *for you*.

Part III: The Initiation

9. Unveiling the Sacred Heart of *Real* Feminine Power: This is the portion of your metamorphosis where you and your "old" life become completely unrecognizable. You struggle with immense fear and doubt, addictions resurface, and the power of your inner darkness begins to overpower your light. Invite in the "Dakini principle" of magic and uncertainty to tip the scale away from death and toward rebirth. Stay with the process and surrender to the Mother Goddess. Die fully to your past self and your ego's plan for your life. In the burial ground of your own sacred heart, let go 100 percent or die.

Part IV: The Ascent

10. Turning On Your Brights: The light starts pouring back in, and you're ready for your resurrection. You commune with your ecstatic nature, learn to "be the lover" in every situation, and step into your *real* edge, your Golden Shadow.

11. Marrying the Divine Masculine: Now you'll find true integration by distinguishing between the Patriarch and the Divine Masculine. By activating Father Love to heal your relationship with the masculine, inner and outer, you create the structures and boundaries needed to protect your vulnerable, feminine core. Through this, you experience the Sacred Marriage and become a sovereign Virgin, able to skillfully activate both masculine and feminine energies.

12. Birthing Your Beautiful Life: When you unearth the genius of your magical, inner child, you open to your innate creative potential, and dream a new dream for your life. After calling upon your inner family to cultivate harmony and cohesion in enacting it, you open to receive the blessings and celebration of a successful journey.

> *Part V: The Homecoming*
>
> **13. Becoming a Whole and Holy Heroine:** Here, it's your turn to test your insight by returning to your roots and serving your family and community. We also meet an inspiring role model who embodies the full spectrum of our journey — from psychological wholeness to spiritual freedom. Last, we remember our ultimate homecoming: full realization of our essential nature and union with the Feminine Face of God, beyond gender, concepts, space, and time.

The Archetype of the Father's Daughter

One evening when I was ten years old, I sat in my white eyelet nightgown at the kitchen table with my father. In front of us, we spread my fourth-grade report card out on the white-and-blue-checked tablecloth. I proudly pointed out all the "excellents" checked off — from reading to math to music to handwriting. In celebration, he pulled a crisp twenty-dollar bill out of his leather wallet and handed it to me, a rare moment of connection for us both. A near-orphan from Minnesota who worked his way up to earn an Ivy League scholarship and then a high-paying job in Manhattan, my father had also always been a straight-A student. He transformed his life from rags to riches by focusing on the one thing he could control — his ambition. I inherited a love of learning from my dad, as well as my immense drive and ambition to succeed, both of which I still value greatly.

But these gifts came with a price. Growing up, I continued to follow in his footsteps. From the fourth-grade "excellents," to high school "high honors," to Ivy League Phi Beta Kappa and summa cum laude, I built my identity and self-worth on the recognition I received through my scholarly success, along with my thin, pretty appearance. I knew that, no matter how lost and insecure I felt inside, as long as I looked good and did well in school, I would receive the love and validation from the world that I so desperately longed for. I later realized that for the first two decades of my life, even though my father, typical of many men of his generation, often traveled and worked long hours away from home, I was my Father's Daughter. I internalized the linear, results-oriented model of patriarchal success that he embodied so well, to enable myself to survive first in my family of origin and later in the world.

Most of us are Father's Daughters, although not always in the same way. Maybe we had fathers who were physically present, but often domineering, aggressive, or even abusive. Or we might have had fathers whom we viewed as too weak and passive, so we aimed ourselves toward becoming the exact opposite. Maybe we had amicable relationships with our fathers and were "Daddy's Little Girls." If we didn't receive enough attention from our fathers, we became "armored amazons," fending for ourselves to get our needs met — and thus becoming Father's Daughters in a roundabout way. As Maureen Murdock explains,

> The armor protects [us] positively insofar as it helps [us] develop professionally and enables [us] to have a voice in the world of affairs, but insofar as the armor shields [us] from [our] own feminine feelings and [our] soft side, [we] tend to become alienated from [our] own creativity, from healthy relationships with men, and from the spontaneity and vitality of living in the moment.[5]

It's no coincidence that most of the women who are drawn to undertake the Heroine's Journey also fall into the archetype of Father's Daughters, and that the first stage of our journey requires that we shed this identity. We've built our selfhoods around being good girls and succeeding at all costs according to deranged masculine principles. As a result, we're tormented by the belief that we need to be extraordinary in order to validate our existence. At some point (or usually many points) along our life journeys, we've felt that who we are at the core is bad. To hide our rotten interiors, we squashed and squelched our inner femininity, while grooming and starving our outer, shapely shells. Some part of us rejected the feminine as distrustful. Our vulnerable, feminine centers withered and withdrew, feeling unloved, unseen, and uncared for by those around us, and we looked to our fathers for love, safety, approval, and recognition. We became Father's Daughters.[6]

What's an Archetype?

C.G. Jung, a Swiss psychiatrist and psychotherapist who founded an-alytical psychology in the first half of the twentieth century, developed the concept of archetypes, along with many other terms that are central to our journey here, such as *the collective unconscious, individuation* (a central process of human development that integrates the opposites), and *extraversion* and *introversion*.

Archetypes are aspects of the collective unconscious that appear in dreams, mythology, and fairy tales as recurring images, patterns, and symbols. They remain hidden (thus unconscious) until they enter our awareness and manifest as behavior and experience at both the indi-vidual and cultural levels. Simultaneously personal and impersonal, ar-chetypes are psycho-spiritual patterns, and certain archetypes activate to organize and influence our thoughts and behaviors. Each stage of life is governed by a new set of archetypes. Mother, Father, Goddess, God, Hero, Heroine, Child, Shadow, Maiden, and Crone are examples of ar-chetypes that can arise within us and help us embody previously unex-pressed aspects of ourselves.

Viewing this archetype from yet another perspective, on a larger, cul-tural scale, we are *all* the daughters of a collective, cultural, all-pervasive pathological father — the Patriarchy. Due to this overarching cultural milieu, which prioritizes dominance, coercion, and power, at this time in history, we are *all* Patriarchy's daughters. We *all* exhaust ourselves to do more, do it better, get ahead, and not be seen as weak or lazy. To function within such overdrive, we bury our intuition, crush our desires, and stomp over our bodies' subtle signals for rest and true nourishment. In driving ourselves so hard, not only do we make ourselves sick and exhausted, but also we hammer the nails into our own coffins of unhappiness. We wonder things like:

"Why do I always feel like I'm behind?"

"Why do I always feel so tired?"

"Why do I feel so disconnected from myself?"

"Why does my life feel so out of balance?"

When we fail to bring the archetype of the Father's Daughter that we all carry inside into the light of our awareness, we prevent a key part of ourselves (like my ten-year-old self in her nightgown) from growing up. She remains wounded and in the driver's seat of our lives, unbeknownst to us!

As daughters of the Patriarchy, we all arrive right here, in this *exact* moment, together. We are at the point where, as grown women, we recognize the need to stop pushing ourselves forward from a hidden agenda to be loved. We wake up to the truth that this pursuit is hollow and perilous. If we don't bring that lifelong, misguided ambition into conscious awareness, we're going to end up driving our dreams — and ourselves — into the ground.

This is what almost happened to one of my students, Catherine. On the outside, she seemed to be doing everything right. She was running a successful women's coaching practice, was happily married to a doting husband, had nurtured a good nest egg of investments, and owned her own home right near her favorite place — the beach. Then some confounding health challenges led her to plunge back into a familiar depression. That's when she reached out to me for mentoring.

"Sara, it's just that I feel like such a..." she sighed, voice trembling, during our first session.

"It's okay, take your time."

"I...I feel like such a hypocrite," she let out, followed by what I sensed was a full-body sob. "Oh my god," she continued, a few sniffles later. "It feels so good just to tell the truth. I didn't realize how much I needed to stop fighting the truth."

Catherine went on to explain that these very funks were what led her to become a coach in the first place. She wanted nothing more than to help other women weather these very challenges. Now, with the resurgence of this debilitating demon, none of Catherine's old tools were working. The more she tried to climb out of her dark well, the more she spiraled down. She began to question her knowledge and integrity.

"I just want to be normal again!" she proclaimed, trying to regain her composure. "Why isn't anything working? What am I doing *wrong*?"

"Catherine," I cut in, "being normal isn't the point. It's not even possible. You're doing absolutely nothing wrong. This is exactly where you need to be."

I knew from my own journey that the real reason Catherine had come to me was far deeper and more beautiful than to regain her status quo.

"This is a *huge* blessing," I continued. "This isn't a setback. It's the bridge to your new life. You know, that one? The one you've always wanted?"

We laughed together for a moment before diving in.

I've mentored hundreds of women like Catherine who have gone through similar rites of passage: midlife crises, "nervous breakdowns" and "spiritual depressions," career shifts, postpartum depressions, miscarriages, the death of a parent or spouse. When things fall apart, we think it's because we've done something wrong. All will be right again if we can just clean ourselves up, rewind, and return to "normal." When we harbor the false belief that life should always be cheerful and challenge-free, *of course* we're going to beat ourselves up when the reality of our lives fails to match our ideals. *I should have saved more money. I shouldn't be feeling this way. I should have more willpower. I should be more confident. I should be able to handle this. I should have appreciated her more when she was alive. I should have, I should have, I should have!*

Serving so many women in crisis shows me again and again how much *every* woman needs to normalize her hardships far more than her false sense of comfy stability. The Buddha taught that "life is suffering." This doesn't mean we're doomed to dwell in misery; rather, this honest perspective empowers us to look at the nature of life head-on. Bumps in the road aren't anomalies. They're unavoidable actualities of being human. We *all* experience them. We *need* to experience them. They signal us to step up and meet the lives that are ours to meet.

As Catherine's story demonstrates, you can never choose when, where, or how your life will call you forth to become a Heroine. There's never a good time for chaos to scramble the tidy package of your life.

Ready or not, your Heroine's Journey always comes to find you through the wise messenger in your depths, your SHE.

Your SHE, Your Feminine Soul

Your feminine soul, which I call your SHE, contains your deepest source of personal power, inner wisdom, and authentic expression. An emanation of the Divine Feminine, SHE allows you to belong to yourself fully, while also being connected to the Sacred All. The direct link between your body, psyche, and divine nature, SHE is both as unique as your fingerprint and as universal as the breath of life. SHE makes every woman a mystic, bridging your personhood and your divinity. When you learn to live in relationship with Her, you harness your latent capacity to be an alchemist, cocreating with the divine to manifest gold out of lead and heaven on earth.

How does this work, exactly? For most of human history, philosophers and mystics pointed out that there are three key aspects of reality: matter, soul, and spirit. Let's take a quick look at each.

Matter is our gross, physical reality (relative). It includes our bodies, trees, mountains, oceans, and so forth — all that we can experience through our five senses.

Spirit is transcendent reality (Absolute). It's what religions and spiritual traditions teach.

Soul is the bridge between matter and spirit. Soul infuses spirit into matter — heaven into earth, divine into human, goddess into woman.

We spend so much of our lives focusing solely on our material realities, forgetting that we are all carry a spark of the divine within us, that most of us never come to truly know our souls. *Yet true healing, wisdom, evolution, joy, and freedom come from expressing your soul's truths in all of your thoughts, words, and actions.* Your soul is the part of you that's old and wise and that came here to experience life through and as you, in order to bring more love and happiness to the world.

This is how some women in our SHE School community speak about their SHEs:

- SHE is the divine and enduring strength of my soul.
- SHE's that "still, small voice" inside of me.
- SHE speaks to me through my intuition and "gut feelings."
- SHE knows what suffering I need to endure to grow and will help to cradle me when it all becomes too much.
- If I can stay grounded and connected with my SHE, I find the fears float away and I'm simply learning another language of love.
- There's no blueprint for where I am at or where I'm going...just my SHE guiding me.

Warning: Be careful not to abstract your SHE. SHE is not an entity outside of you. *SHE is you* — the deepest, wisest, most divine part of you, trying to take root in your unique body and personality structure. SHE is your True Self (with a capital *S*).

Here's how Maggie, one of the women in our community, voiced this recognition:

> I now realize that my SHE is just me, and is not going to communicate with me in a way that seems to come from outside myself. And I realize that I've always been looking for the divine far outside of myself. I expected it to be this huge knock over the head and I guess the idea that it was me didn't seem good enough, which I suppose goes to some subconscious belief that I am not good enough. It is a really profound realization for me. SHE is me, just that. And all that as well. Beautiful and momentous at the same time!

This Is an Initiation

Sweet sixteen, your first period, the loss of your virginity, marriage, birth, your fiftieth birthday — as women we know such outer initiations well. They serve as milestones of growth. Our communities and families honor us during some of these commencements. Others we acknowledge alone.

In all cases, most initiations today stand shallow and empty. They no longer carry the rich, magical ritual they once did. Rites of passage seem to be luxuries in our busy lives, so we hurry through them. Even worse: sometimes we don't take the time to celebrate at all. *Why take time for me,* we ask? *That's selfish. I have too many other things to do right now.*

In our rush, we forget that our lives are a series of initiations. Women's health pioneer Dr. Christiane Northrup uses the metaphor of passing through a series of wombs over the course of our lives.[7] Each stage gives birth to the next. Let's stop rushing back to work mere days after giving birth or burying a loved one. Let's acknowledge that even if we're not visibly bleeding or injured, we sometimes have inner wounds and illnesses that require time, *lots* of time, to heal. Feminine wisdom blossoms within us, and on this planet, through this very process of passing from womb to womb — death to rebirth. Our initiations help all of humanity to evolve and therefore demand our respect and loving presence.

As an initiation, this book is here to give you all the tools and inspiration you need to face yourself and your life — full-on. It is here to urge you forward, into the chaos, the mess, and the uncertainty. It is here to roar at you when you whimper and want to turn back. It is here to cradle you when all you need is the Mother's mercy. It is here to protect you when you face the inner demons that you fear might destroy you. It is here to sing to you when you arrive in the field of your own forgiveness.

Please, Don't Be a Voyeur

Before we go any further, I need to send out a blast of fierce love. So many of us would rather live our lives on the sidelines, watching or reading about someone else's Heroine's Journey. Too many of us think we don't have what it takes to embark on the journey ourselves. If you're reading this, commit here and now to *not* be a sideline sitter! This is within your reach. You can do this! *Anyone* can do this. The only way to fail is to not answer the call.

Like the famous scene in *Eat, Pray, Love* where Elizabeth Gilbert lies sobbing on her bathroom floor with the realization that she must end her marriage, we too have received that middle of the night call (and have also ended up a slobbering mess in the bathroom).[8] The quest always starts with those questions whimpered in the dark: *What is my life really about? Why am I really here?*

Sure, we can wake up the next morning and put frozen spoons on our eyes to hide the swelling. We can walk the dog, make our coffee, and resume our life as if nothing ever happened. We can either ignore the call or pursue it. Just know that you will pay a huge price if you choose the former. You will die, bit by bit, if you don't listen to the call; for when you don't answer the call, you don't listen to your SHE's desire to come home to your Self. If you don't choose growth, your soul will stop trying to get your attention and you *will* eventually *actually* die. From that perspective, we don't really have a choice, do we?

On this journey, success means living from — not just listening to — your inner wisdom (your SHE) and rolling with the punches of whatever that brings. Along this journey there are no shortcuts. There are no hiding places. It requires your full participation. You have to face every single part of yourself and your life in order to proceed to the next step. To become a Heroine you need to melt all the places within you that have been frozen and cut off from the support of the Great Mother. You need to reconnect all the parts of your inner landscape that have been disharmonious for so long.

Only you can do this. The Heroine's Journey has no "exit" — and that's a good thing. Because on the other side of this journey is...*you*. Not the "you" that you are right now, but the "you" you've not yet scripted. The courageous you who has created with gusto and humility in partnership with your eternal soul the life you most want to live.

If you're feeling some trepidation, that's a good sign. We all need to get a little scared by the level of responsibility that this kind of journey demands! Here's the good news: even though we'll each undergo our initiations alone, we'll walk the path together, one step at a time.

Journaling Questions

- What are the biggest life crises you've experienced? What did you learn from each of these, and how did they change you?
- How have you defined success in your life? How did your parents, caretakers, teachers, and role models define success? What might be a truer definition of success for you now?
- In what ways are you a Father's and/or Patriarchy's Daughter? How have you pushed yourself to meet external definitions of success in order to be seen, appreciated, and loved? How has this impacted you, both positively and negatively?
- What emergent female role models and archetypes can give you more confidence as you take some steps along this new path?

Chapter 2

Entering Your
Inner House

Some people say home is where you come from,
but I think it's a place you need to find,
like it's scattered and you pick pieces of it up along the way.

— Katie Kacvinsky, *Awaken*

It's time to learn how to take care of yourself. I mean *really* take care of yourself. The most profound self-care practice we can do is right under our noses. It's an *internal* practice, so simple and obvious that we often completely miss it. When we bypass this step, no amount of external pampering can nourish our depths when we're feeling depleted, afraid, overwhelmed, or insufficient.

Self-care is just this: lovingly meeting ourselves exactly where we are and allowing things to be as they are. When we can hold ourselves in this way, our inner world starts to become softer, gentler. We start to trust our own basic goodness, and we even come to learn that irritation, aversion, doubt, and resistance aren't to be evicted through our self-care; they're to be allowed and included by it.

Devoid of our loving presence, our bodies become more like haunted houses than goddess temples. How did we end up this way? Trauma has frozen inside. Our bodies house all of our old memories, sensations, thoughts, and emotions. Scary, unpredictable, too much, too little: At some point in our lives, our bodies became scary to inhabit. They craved foods that make us fat, sex that makes us "bad," or pleasure that makes us "selfish." They grew hair in inconvenient places. They bled through our pants and stained our sheets.

Deep down in our bodies' depths roam the ghosts of unhealed trauma, abandoned creative passions, sensual desires, intuition, and the true power that comes from who we *are*, rather than what we *do*. Our bodies aren't indentured servants here to labor for us until we take our dying breath. They are sacred chalices, home to our SHEs. The chalice, a metaphor for the Divine Feminine, is the lake, bowl, vessel, womb, or grail. We are not only embodied as but also governed by circles. Within this roundness, we house the entire universe — each season of the sun, sea, earth, and moon. We are microcosmic containers within which the miracle of life can grow, flourish, and decay. Our bodies help us live out the unique contribution we're each here to make in the short time that we have. Our bodies *always* tell the truth and hold the information we need to thrive.

The confusion we harbor about our embodiment has reached epidemic proportions. We're all living in a time that values spirit (masculine) over matter (feminine). These two qualities exist in everything and are independent of gender. Each man holds feminine, or yin, qualities, just as each woman holds masculine, or yang, qualities — in different degrees. When we appropriately balance these two poles, we become integrated human beings.

The well-known yin/yang symbol from Taoism illustrates how the coessential polarities of masculine and feminine energies intermingle and flow together to create a balanced whole. Yin is inside, slow, passive, dim, downward, female, moon, while yang is outside, rapid, active, bright, upward, male, sun.

Masculine awareness ascends. It rises up and out of the body, seeking spaciousness and the bird's-eye view (think meditation, quantum physics, and the compartmentalization and mechanization of "the body" in Western medicine). Feminine awareness descends. It moves down and into the body, all the way into the heart of the earth (think belly dancing, Mother Teresa kissing lepers in the slums of Calcutta, and the use of medicine spirits in plants to heal the body). Ultimately, we need both to truly thrive as individuals, and as a society. We need both dancing *and* sitting still, penicillin *and* echinacea, splitting the atom *and* activating our compassionate hearts.

Since we've all inadvertently prioritized the "up and out" (masculine) current, we need to remember how to go "down and in" — not just as a concept, but as a felt experience. When we inhabit our bodies, we feel like we've come home. Embodying our womanhood needs to be a full-time affair.

The Holy Trinity in Your Body

Every house holds different layers — the foundation, frame, wiring, walls, insulation, and interior. The same holds true for the houses of our bodies. We harbor three main layers. Each needs to be addressed on our journeys to embodying our SHEs.

1. Gross: This is the "matter" layer that we discussed in chapter 1. We can see this with our eyes and feel it with our hands. It contains our organs, bones, muscles, tissues, and circulatory system.

2. Subtle: This is the "soul/SHE" layer we explored in chapter 1. Composed of our thoughts and feelings, we experience our subtle body as our "felt sense." It's also called the *inner* or *energy* body, and ancient lineages in yoga and martial arts teach that *prana* or *chi* carry vital life force through invisible energy pathways in the subtle body (called *nadis* or *meridians*). Containing the most unrecognized and underdeveloped parts of our bodies, the subtle layer holds our childhood memories, ancestral wounding and wisdom, as well as our potential to fully embody our soul's purpose. Unfelt experiences in our subtle bodies create physical tensions and illnesses. Our subtle body serves as the bridge between human and divine, psychology and spirituality. Real healing and transformation happen when we learn to palpate and participate with our subtle bodies.

3. Causal: This is the "spirit" layer. Spirit animates and gives life to our bodies each time we breathe. We can't make ourselves breathe, for we're always *being* breathed. Our lives begin with an inhalation and end with an exhalation. The more we heal our lifelong wounds by inhabiting the dark, dusty corners of our gross and subtle layers, the more freely we can breathe, and the more fully we fill ourselves with the presence of the divine.

Melting Your Inner Ice Ceiling

When we start to stretch our awareness south of our breasts, we encounter our first obstacle: the icy sheaths over our power centers. Yogic traditions call this seat of our personal power our third chakra. *Chakra* means "wheel" or "turning" in Sanskrit and serves as one of seven meeting points for the currents of life force energy that run through us, connecting spirit with matter. Western anatomy calls the third chakra our solar plexus, or the confluence of nerves right above the center of our diaphragm, between our lowest ribs.

We have three main energy centers in the fronts of our bodies, our bellies, solar plexuses, and chests. Each of these opens and closes like a camera shutter in response to external stimuli. When they're closed, we feel guarded and shut down. When they're open, we feel alive, receptive, and in love with all of life.

We'll work with all three of these energy centers during our journey, for our aim is to cultivate such deep self-understanding that we know exactly where, when, why, and how we close — and can remain open at all costs. In this chapter we're focusing on the first two energy centers only — our solar plexus and belly. Let's look at our solar plexus first.

The solar plexus freezes up when we don't feel seen or met by those around us. It closes when we feel overcome by more emotions than we have the inner or outer resources to handle and, as a result, either withdraw or react. Both responses undermine our personal power.

Our power centers lock down when we feel unsafe and don't know how to adequately self-soothe. Frozen over, we're sure to stay out of harm's way by keeping our voices rooted in our intellect, rather than in the wild soil of our belly. After decades of shutting down, we're met with gaping silence when the day finally comes and we find the courage to ask ourselves, "What do I really want here? What do I truly desire? What's the voice of my soul?"

Anna, one of the women in the SHE School, wrote about her experience with this in our private online forum.

> Whenever people ask "What are your dreams? What do you want to manifest in the world?" I have always been a bit uncomfortable. I realized this week that I truly don't have a dream(s). Everything I have done or accomplished or worked toward has been as a result of my perfectionism and my deep-rooted fear of not being loved if I am not perfect or productive. Things that look like they would be dreams if others were judging were truly only done from this unauthentic place in me.
>
> What was interesting is that as I processed this I wondered if I would feel really, really empty, but I didn't. I just sat with the realization and felt into my body. And I asked… "What do I want?" And I started to feel something deep in my solar plexus. Just a feeling, not even words to describe it except that it felt "full," and so I just said thanks and felt into it. For the rest of the week, I used that as my guide — just feeling into that place, especially when I got too much into my head and started trying to think my way out.

As Anna's experience so beautifully demonstrates, re-scripting our lives — our greatest creative undertaking — begins in our *internal* landscapes. Inside our bodies, we clear out the ancestral memories that have been unconsciously running our lives. We devise a new, inner road map by etching out fresh cellular pathways between our heads, hearts, solar plexuses, and bellies. To let the old stories and self-identities go and free our voices to speak what's ours to speak, we need to unfreeze and inhabit the parts of our bodies that our SHEs' voices need to take root in in order to be heard.

A few years ago I booked a bodywork session with a local healer to help me with this process. At the start of the session, I lay down naked, covered, and faceup on the massage table. The healer stood behind my head. Barefoot, she placed her warm hands on my diaphragm, just at the base of my rib cage.

"Breathe into my hands," she instructed, "try to push me off of you."

Inhale. Exhale.

"Breathe into your side body."

Inhale.

She paused and waited for my next exhalation, sliding her hands firmly down from my diaphragm, in toward my waist.

"Keep wiggling your hips," she instructed, "like a belly dancer. Good. That's it! Now, wiggle your toes, stretch your legs. Press out through your heels."

As I followed her instructions, together we danced around the throbbing warmth in my solar plexus. Again. And again.

"Now, on your exhale make a sound. Open and close your jaw. Imagine an unraveling from your solar plexus, all the way up your throat and to the base of your tongue. Feel all of that becoming free."

"Ahhhhhhh." I moaned a low growl that ended with a tentative crackle. My core tightened again from the awkwardness of hearing my own raw voice in the room for the first time.

My session with the healer reinforced my awareness of my weakest link. Every time I had something to say but didn't, my solar plexus collapsed. Every time I took an action that betrayed my inner authority, my solar plexus ached. Every time I squirmed away from, rather than lovingly met, my fear, self-doubt, or sadness, my solar plexus tightened into a knot of unmet needs.

Your Inner Ice Ceiling can't be shattered. It must be loved. You can't experience feminine power without this step, because your SHE must span the great divide from your head to your belly in order to embody your divine potential. You must breathe into your solar plexus until it melts into its intrinsic, vulnerable pulsation. This is an organic process that unfolds for each of us in different ways. But this is how you begin to let Her all the way *in* and *down*.

Breathing into Your Inner Ice Ceiling

1. Bring the palms of your hands to your rib cage, fingers pointing inward until your middle fingers touch.

2. Feel the heels of your hands cupping the sides of your ribs.

3. Breathe into your hands, trying to push your hands outward to each side of you as you inhale.

4. When you exhale, gently put some pressure on your ribs until your middle fingers meet again.

5. Try that two more times. Each time, allow your breath to become fuller, without overstraining.

6. After your third exhale, bring your awareness back into your middle fingers. Gently press them into the soft space between your lowest ribs, which is called your xiphoid process.

7. Continue to lovingly massage this space with your fingertips. Inhale and exhale fully, noticing whatever you feel here — physically and emotionally.

8. Remove your hands and lovingly breathe into this newly tenderized space. Fully welcome any lingering sensations.

9. Throughout your day, especially during stressful moments, practicing breathing into your solar plexus.

Your True Home in Your Belly

In 2000, I attended my first ten-day silent Buddhist meditation retreat at a forest monastery in southern Thailand. I sat cross-legged on a ragged maroon meditation cushion, among about fifty other foreigners. Ajan Poh, the bony, seventy-five-year-old head abbot who sat perched on a wooden platform in front of us all, seemed to float effortlessly inside his saffron robes. After a too-long stretch of sweaty silence, he leaned his wrinkled lips toward the microphone.

"Breathe in. Breathe out."

His voice crackled through the humid air, amid calls of cicadas and roosters.

"Rest your attention in your belly," he instructed slowly. "When your mind wanders, bring it back to your belly."

All spiritual traditions have some version of these instructions. Rest your attention in your belly center — two inches below your navel and above your pubic bone, just forward of your spine. The Japanese call it the *hara*; the Chinese, the *dantien*; the Hindus, the second chakra (or *Svadisthana*, which in Sanskrit means "one's true home"). These ancients understood that our belly houses our intuitive center and our internal fountain of youth. Scientists now understand that our "second brain" lives in our belly, measuring about nine meters end to end from the esophagus to the anus and comprised of 100 million neurons (more than either the spinal cord or the peripheral nervous system). Responsible for more than merely digestion and elimination, this "second brain" informs our state of mind and emotional well-being. Ninety-five percent of the body's serotonin, the "feel-good" hormone involved in preventing depression and regulating sleep, appetite, and body temperature, is produced in the colon. Our belly houses our "gut instincts," communicating feelings up from the vagus nerve to the brain whenever there's an external threat.[1]

Even though our belly brains evolved before the brains in our heads, and poor belly health is now linked as a cause of autism, depression, multiple sclerosis, osteoporosis, Alzheimer's, and Parkinson's (to name a few conditions), we still don't trust the power of our bellies![2] We scurry around "uptight," "in our head," afraid or simply too busy to feel what's going on down below. For most of the day, we're drawn out of our bodies, eyes glued to colorful screens. In the United States, where women are still recovering from the spell of Puritanical notions like "the lower body is the devil," we're afraid of the unpredictable messiness of our rage, grief, lust, and power — all of which reside in our bellies. When we ignore the "butterflies" in our stomachs, we're more likely to reach for the box of cookies, the cigarette, or the glass of wine. Onward we rush through the world, ignoring the weariness and the whine of our bodies.

It's time to put into action what all spiritual traditions point to as the most preliminary (and advanced) practice, and what Western science now backs up. When we honor the wisdom that lives in our intuitive belly centers, we learn to find a sense of inner safety and "home" there.

Connecting to the Earth

In order to connect with ourselves, we need to first connect to the earth. This process, called *earthing*, stands as one of the most important self-care practice we can do each day. When we're cut off from the earth, we're also cut off from our bodies, and then we can't hear our inner wisdom telling us what we need to do next. We're disconnected from our greatest inner resource — our embodied sense of home and wholeness.

Once again, scientific studies now tout what sages have known for centuries — there are tremendous physical benefits to earthing. Simply putting our bare feet on the ground outside for ten to twenty minutes a day helps to reduce chronic inflammation, the primary cause of virtually all diseases. Since our skin serves as a conductor, when we touch any part of our skin to the earth, free electrons — the most powerful antioxidants available — flow from the earth into our bodies. Clinical studies have shown grounding experiments to cause beneficial changes in heart rate, decreased skin resistance, and decreased levels of inflammation.[3]

Earthing also helps to placate us emotionally and mentally by shifting our nervous system out of a stress response and into its parasympathetic, or "rest and digest," mode. Just as crying babies calm down when we hold them, we too calm down when we feel held. Since it's not always possible for another human being to hold us, we have to extend our awareness to what is already *always* holding us — the earth herself.

When it's warm enough here in Colorado, I love practicing yoga barefoot in my backyard. If I'm in the throes of a busy day and feeling scattered, I'll simply take a ten-minute break from my workday. I go outside, take off my shoes and socks, stand on the grass in a patch of sunlight, and do the visualization I offer next. I always return to my desk feeling more energized, relaxed, and in touch with my inner resources.

Earth and Belly Breathing

To partake in a meditation to connect to the earth, go to www.TheBookof SHE.com/practices, where you can listen to an audio file that will guide you through this visualization. I've also included it in written form here.

First, close your eyes, pause, and notice how centered and earthy you feel. Don't change anything. Rate yourself on a scale from one to ten — one being completely scattered and anxious and ten being fully present and at home in yourself. Speak (or whisper) aloud the number that feels accurate. Don't think too much about it. Trust your first thought. There's no right or wrong answer. Good. Remember that number. We'll come back to it.

Now we'll begin the practice. Sit or stand with your feet on the floor or earth, hip-distance apart, outer edges parallel. Now, relax your feet. Unclench your toes. Feel as if the skin on the tops and bottoms of your feet is stretching, widening into the earth. If you're standing up, place your hands on your lower belly. Let your thumbs touch on your navel, your index fingers on your pubic bone, forming a diamond shape between your hands. If you're sitting down and that hand position feels uncomfortable, rest your hands, faceup, on the tops of your thighs.

Close your eyes. Close your mouth, and rest the tip of your tongue softly on your upper palate, behind your upper row of teeth. Breathe softly through your nose, allowing your inhales and exhales to become equal in length and intensity. Allow yourself to feel like you're "being breathed" rather than controlling your breath.

Now imagine that there's a golden thread falling down from the ceiling or sky. It passes through the crown of your head, your upper palette, center of your throat, heart, and diaphragm. Through the center of your pelvic floor, and descends down into the earth right between your feet. Envision this golden thread, trusting whatever you feel or notice. Now, sense where along this thread your attention feels like it's resting right now. Trust your first instinct about this. Wherever your attention's located, watch it descend down the golden thread until it rests right in the center of your belly. If your attention was already resting in your belly, let it remain there.

Envision now that all of your awareness is located about two inches below your navel, two inches above your pubic bone, and two inches in front of your spine. You can also envision that your entire head has traveled down the golden thread and temporarily lives in your belly. Breathe into your belly center now. If your hands are resting on your abdomen, let them swell forward as you breathe in and contract back toward your spine as you breathe out. If and when thoughts arise, release them and return to the spaciousness of your belly center.

Now, keep part of your attention resting in your belly center and extend the other half of your attention down into the center of the earth. Feel the qualities of the earth in the part of the world you're in beneath you — the exact season and attributes. Let each inhale extend all the way down into the core of the earth. Stay here for several breaths.

With your next inhalation, envision that you're drawing energy up from the center of the earth, through the soles of your feet, up your leg bones, in through the base of your body, and into your belly center. On your exhalation, store the earth's medicine here. If you're a visual person, notice the color of the earth energy that you're drawing up. Inhale, draw it up and in; exhale, store it in your belly for future fuel when you need more grounding or energy.

Now imagine that there's an earthing cord descending from your tailbone down into the center of the earth. Notice how thick and strong the cord is. Does it seem more like a waterfall or a rope? Clearly see each end of the cord — one attaching firmly to the center of the earth, the other end to the base of your spine. See the energy of the earth rising up from this grounding cord into your body as you inhale. As you exhale, circulate it anywhere in your body that needs it. If you're feeling really scattered, ask to increase the flow of earth energy up your earthing cord by 50 or even 100 percent.

Take at least several more breaths in this way, staying as long as you need to until you feel filled by the earth's strong, grounded presence

To complete, rest your attention back in your belly center. Feel your body from the tips of your toes to the crown of your head. Notice what it feels like to ground yourself. Now, slowly open your eyes.

Keeping your hands on your belly, take a few steps around the room, keeping your attention in your belly.

Once again, just as we did at the beginning, without changing anything, notice how grounded you feel. Rate yourself on a scale from one to ten — one being completely scattered and anxious and ten being fully present and at home in yourself. Once you arrive at your number, compare this to how you rated yourself at the start of this meditation. How has this earthing practice changed your experience of yourself? Feel the answer inside your body. You don't need to find words for it. Just sense it and get familiar with the lived experience of being grounded.

Advanced practice: Return to your belly awareness as often as you can during the day. Place your hands on your belly from time to time and check in — what's happening in your belly now? This is your intuitive, feeling center. Notice what information you're receiving.

Practice connecting with your belly when you're talking, listening, at your computer, or driving. Ancient adepts taught that the more we can keep our attention in our bellies, the more energy and vitality we'll have. Constantly getting lost in thought and external stimuli depletes our precious energy reserves. Once again, instead of always reaching for caffeine or other pick-me-ups for energy, practice this long-term energy preservation as often as you remember to.

One of the many wonderful advantages of the practice of earthing is that you can do it anytime, anywhere. You don't need a patch of grass to do it! I did it when I waited for the teakettle to boil this morning and when I sat down at my desk to write. You can do it in the shower, even while waiting in line at a café. If you want to test yourself to see whether or not you've shifted your center of gravity from your head to your belly center, lift up one foot and close your eyes. If you can balance, you're in your belly.

It's empowering to recognize that the earth lives within you, always. Upon learning this exercise, Adrianne, one of the sisters in the SHE School, observed,

> I always associated earthing with my feet growing roots down to the earth only. It was very helpful to know that grounding comes *from* our belly. When I pinpointed the spot, it made all the sense in the world! I think for most of my life when I felt that rumble or sinking feeling in my belly, I thought I was hungry, so I just ate something. Now I see that in those cases what I'm really hungry for is a grounded connection to myself.

Like Adrianne, when you pause to actually feel your belly, you're able to give yourself the deeper kind of nourishment that it's usually asking for.

Cultivating an Inner Sense of "Home"

When first learning to feel at home within ourselves, we need calm, soothing environments to help us get grounded. In the SHE School, I asked women what helps them to feel like they're "home." Here are some of their responses:

- Walking outside among the trees
- Camping and sleeping outside
- My meditation cushion
- My yoga practice
- Playing with my nieces and nephews
- Cuddling with my dog
- Watching a movie in bed
- My husband's chicken soup
- Swimming in the ocean

There's nothing complicated about any of these things. Most are available to us every day. The more we immerse ourselves in these outer safe refuges, the more we're able to mirror them inwardly. Then when we find ourselves feeling like we're falling through the air with nothing to take hold of (as will always be the case during our initiations), we're able to more easily cultivate a sense of ground within the only steady refuge we ever have — our own bodies.

Your Body as Your Inner House

This is an adaptation of a visualization created by my friend and colleague Jill Satterfield, founder of Vajra Yoga + Meditation.[4] Please visit www.TheBookofSHE.com/practices to listen to and download an audio file that will guide you through this visualization. I've also included it in written form here.

Come to a comfortable seated position, either sitting in a chair, or on a cushion on the floor. Rest your hands, palms facing down on your thighs. Extend your spine up toward the ceiling as you feel your hips and legs remaining heavy. Gently close your eyes and relax your face and mouth. Without changing anything, find your natural, relaxed breath.

Be childlike — open, curious, a little playful. As images arise in your imagination, don't censor them. Remember that the first image you see usually arises from your intuition. First thought, best thought.

Now, feel your torso. Feel your entire torso — front, back, left and right sides. Feel the entire length, width, and circumference of your torso, from your pelvic floor all the way up to the top of your neck. Feel as much of it as you can, all at once.

Envision this space, from your torso to your neck, as a house. Your house — the one you've lived in since the moment you were born, and the one you'll live in until you die. What does your house look like? Is it a mud hut, an urban brownstone, sprawling ranch, or something else? See as much of your house as you can. Look closely at the details. What color is it? What's it made out of? What do the doors and windows look like? When we live with something every day of our lives, it can grow very familiar and we stop noticing the details. Take some time here to look closely.

Now let's go inside the house. See yourself walking up the front path and opening the door. Step inside the house. What does it feel like to be in here? What's your first impression of the inside of your house?

Let's take a look around now. What part of the house feels the brightest? Feel the place in your body that feels the brightest. What room feels the most dusty and cluttered? In which room do your parents stay when they come to visit? What about the one that still holds your favorite childhood toys? Which room holds all of your secrets — those things you've never told another soul? Make sure to really pause and feel each area of your body. If you start to get distracted or overwhelmed, come back to your breath in your belly and resume when you feel ready again. Which room needs a good cleaning? Which room is so dark that no one ever goes in it? Which room feels really breezy and comfortable?

Still with your eyes closed, place your hands on the parts of your house that felt the most dark, cluttered, and in need of repair. Feel the love and warmth in the palms of your hands. Notice: Are these areas tighter than others? Do they hold more stress and tension? Are they harder for you to breathe with? Take a moment with your hands on these darker rooms of your house, feeling them exactly as they are.

Next, place your hands on the parts of your house that felt the brightest, most spacious, and comfortable. Notice the qualities of your breath and the tissues in these areas. Keep your hands there, feeling them exactly as they are.

When you feel ready, slowly return your hands to your lap. Feel the breath in your belly, feel the room that you're in from the house of your body, and slowly open your eyes.

The Root of Our Disconnection

A shaman once warned me: "Watch out for anyone who can't keep a plant alive. They are not connected to life and the earth." Her words really stuck with me, because I used to be one of those people. It was only when I was thirty and moved to Boulder that I took on the task of filling my house with plants *and* keeping them alive.

To do so, I had to learn to tend to a life other than my own by attuning to their needs. Did they look wilted? On which days did what plants need watering, and how much? I learned to create a home for them, and in turn, for myself. We became a family, living and thriving together. This was a *huge* step for me. Like many of us, I grew up in a dysfunctional family, where the imprint in my nervous system of unconditional holding, empathy, nourishment, and underlying harmony simply didn't exist. I felt it wasn't safe for me to express my needs, so I learned to ignore them and leave them unmet. This left me feeling anxious, insecure, and unsafe. I then grew up with the underlying belief that the world is unsafe, everyone is a possible threat, and I'm a bad person, undeserving of love and happiness.

Now, as a grown woman, I understand that this self and worldview doesn't serve anyone, and that most of us walk around either consciously or unconsciously feeling this way at some level. We all pass down wounds of not truly seeing or meeting one another from generation to generation, until someone in the family does the inner work required to create a new pattern. As a key part of my healing over the past two decades, I've had to learn how to the create a responsive, loving, safe environment for *myself* that I lacked as a little girl, both internally and externally, just as I did for my plants.

John Welwood, who is one of my teachers and a Buddhist psychotherapist, author, and pioneer in psycho-spiritual inquiry, explains that everything in the universe needs to be held:

> The earth is held in space....DNA is held within cells, and cells are held within the larger tissues and organs of the body. Leaves are held by a tree, trees are held by the dirt. And growing children are held within the family environment.[5]

The same is true for us. We need to feel held within the container of our own loving awareness.

Unfortunately, as young children we all learned to disconnect from both our inner and outer "ground." At some point in our formative years (usually before the age of eight), we all experienced a moment of tremendous openness. Maybe we ripped our clothes off and ran through the kitchen or squealed with joy in the middle of the supermarket. In that moment, our caretakers, most likely because of their own unmet suffering, were not able to receive our innocently uncensored rapture, much less support the vulnerability beneath it. Consequently, we learned that in order to stay safe and be loved, we needed to shut down. We started to view our openness as threatening, so we strived to manage and control it in two primary ways — dissociating and armoring. Layer by layer, we covered over our instinctual natures with self-protective habits. From that point onward the walls between our inner and outer worlds continued to grow stronger and taller

Since our nervous systems weren't fully developed as children, we didn't have the inner tools required to help us process painful experiences when we were young. (Our prefrontal cortex, which enables emotional regulation and more sophisticated rationalization, doesn't start to develop until adolescence, and our brains aren't fully formed until we're at least in our mid-twenties!) Plus, most of us didn't get the empathic care we needed from those around us to process our complex feelings, either. We quickly discovered that it was simply too painful to feel, so we stopped listening to our own wise, internal guidance system. Our feelings, and the needs they pointed to, weren't okay to express, so we gave up even trying. Then, as our feelings revealed themselves through sensations in our body, we cut off from our bodies. The resulting tension created armor and iciness over our vulnerable feelings. How many of us feel tight in our necks, chests, shoulders, and diaphragms? Sure, part of this is a result of our increasingly sedentary lifestyle, but part of it is based in this funda-mental dissociation we experienced as children. When we felt threatened, we shielded our tender hearts and bellies.

Our necks too feel like thick steel cords, because they help to armor the flow of communication between our heads, hearts, and bellies. Our vibrant earth centers have become dark pits of frightening, undigested feelings. As we grow older, it takes more and more energy to keep them there, hidden away from the light of day and our own loving awareness. Through this, we are left feeling empty, separate, anxious, tense, and per-petually lacking. This has become our status quo. Growing up with the cloud of "negative love" over our intrinsic, loving core, we never learned any other way to relate to the world than to take on the negative behaviors of our parents.

This pain has often been passed on between generations, and it will continue unless we choose to follow the path of self-healing. Unless we make changes, we will remain trapped in the ancient pattern of being painfully dissociated from ourselves and others.

It's also essential to realize that we can't heal these parts of ourselves in isolation, solely through external measures. They're *relational* wounds, so we need love, intimacy, and interconnectivity — with ourselves and others — to penetrate such lifelong pain.

As you begin to move forward, remember that you now have two new tools to add to your self-care practice: connecting to the earth and coming home to the earth of your own body. These are the simplest, most overlooked, most profoundly effective self-care practices we can ever engage in as women.

Journaling Questions

- When, where, and why do you feel ungrounded?
- What feels like "home" to you?
- Where do you feel the most tension and armoring in your body? What parts of your body feel numb, shut down, or frozen? What parts feel alive, warm, and safe?
- What do you feel in your belly *right now*? Pause, feel, and notice.

Chapter 3

Healing the Mother Wound

The mother wound is bigger than each of us.

— Dr. Christiane Northrup, *Mother-Daughter Wisdom*

Lama Tsering Everest, a Buddhist teacher, advocates that we must regard everyone we meet as our mother in a past life. The ex who broke your heart. The mangy dogs that chased after me in the back alleys of Thailand. The smelly man who sat next to you on the plane. Everyone. Yet while it's hard to revere our enemies as our mothers, perhaps it's even harder for us to really and truly revere *our actual mothers*. Along with idealizing images of voluptuous, jewel-laden goddesses as the Feminine Divine, let's not forget to cherish the most sacred of *all* female archetypes — the Mother.

Mothers and daughters we all are. So beautiful and complicated! No matter our age, we feel a tangled sense of sanctum and irritation when we think of our mothers. We may proclaim, "I will *never* be anything like my mother!" only to grow up and find ourselves talking, walking, even thinking exactly like her. Rather than viewing this as a bad thing, we need to reframe our relationships with our mothers, seeing them as our most potent allies on the path to wholeness and Awakening.

In Buddhism, such an ally is known as a "spiritual friend." Your life and your Heroine's Journey begin in relationship with your mother. This connection lays the foundation for all your future relationships and for your own felt sense of what it means to be a woman. In order to love yourself as you would your own child, you need to also love your mother.

Without first deeply understanding and healing this firmament of our femininity, no amount of positive affirmation, visualizations, or feel-good techniques can ever deliver us the shining sense of confidence, self-worth, and self-esteem we all so deeply crave. Since low self-esteem lingers as the top grievance for every woman I know and work with, it's well worth it for us to spend some time here. The effects of healing the Mother Wound reverberate into *all* dimensions of our inner and outer lives. Let's go to the root of our self-hatred, for learning to re-mother ourselves is the only thing that can ever heal that.

Mother-Daughter Attunement

Douglas W. Winnicott, a British child psychiatrist in the 1950s, referred to the healing space of the inner and outer "ground" that we explored in the previous chapter as a "holding environment."[1] This holding environment extends beyond just the physical affection all children need to the larger, kindhearted, and empathic atmosphere around the children as well. Like the literal womb, this outer womb provides all the physical, emotional, and psychological sustenance children need in order to grow and thrive in their formative years.

For the 1950s, this was huge. In a time when child-rearing norms urged mothers to let their children cry and to bottle-feed them, Winnicott intervened with a new prescription that he called "the Good Enough Mother." Following this approach, a mother creates an emotional environment where she's interested and available. She stays in the room with her children while they play, she gets up to hold her children when they cry, and she breastfeeds them. Winnicott understood that children *need* their parents to hold them — both physically *and* emotionally.

For young children who have virtually no language skills and zero capacity to even know what a feeling is (much less how to work with one!), their emotional reality colors *everything*. Young children need their parents to help them make sense of their strong emotions through mirroring and attunement. For girls, when a mother attunes to her daughter, she acts like a tuning fork. By being loving and attentive, the mother enables the child to regulate herself through her mother's mood, thus allowing her to shift out of her stress response and into her parasympathetic nervous system.

Emotions around connection may play an even stronger role in little girls than they do in little boys. When I held my niece, Hattie, when she was a baby, she often looked up at me from my arms. Unlike her older brothers, who often looked around the room when I used to hold them, Hattie hooked her gaze intently to mine, mimicking each expression I showered upon her. Louann Brizendine, MD, author of *The Female Brain*, explains, "Baby girls are born interested in emotional expression. They make meaning about themselves from every look, touch, and reaction from the people they come into contact with. From these cues they discover whether they are worthy, lovable, or annoying."[2]

Dr. Edward Tronick's famous "Still Face Experiment" also demonstrated the profound link between the emotions of a mother and her child by filming a mother-daughter pair in two scenarios.[3] In the first one, the mother remains responsive and connected to her child. She smiles, her eyes light up, and she speaks in a playful, singsong voice to her little one. In response, her baby laughs, coos, and "talks" (or babbles) to her mother. In the second scenario, the mother remains completely unresponsive. Her face stays somber, her eyes dull and lifeless. She shows no expression whatsoever. The baby, in turn, desperately tries to get her mother's attention back by smiling, laughing, and pointing to things in the room. As the baby starts to feel more and more distress about her mother's emotional absence, she lets out a high-pitched squeal. Ultimately, she resorts to crying and flailing her limbs to regain her mother's attention.

Babies need their mothers to mirror back to them what they're feeling, and then to interpret it slightly so the child can understand: "It's okay, sweetie. I see you're afraid. Mama's here. I've got you."

Contact and Space

Just a few phrases from a mother to her child (*It's okay, sweetie; I see you're afraid; Mama's here; I've got you*) show us that attunement isn't rocket science. While it's crucial for cultivating an empathic holding environment that allows a child to feel safe and secure in the world, attunement is a very simple process. For attunement to occur, two essential aspects are always present: contact and space.

Contact looks and feels like:

- seeing
- touching
- mirroring
- expressing empathy
- caring
- being attentive
- holding
- acting with kindness

Without contact a child feels abandoned. However, contact alone isn't sufficient. Even infants need to feel they are allowed to be themselves. Children also need *space* in order to cultivate a sense of safety, trust, and ease in the world.

Space looks and feels like:

- generosity
- allowance
- freedom of expression
- trust
- forgiveness

Contact without space quickly becomes intrusive, controlling, claustrophobic, and smothering. On the other hand, contact and space together create attunement, and the felt experience of attunement is a sense of deep, abiding, unconditional joy.

Obviously it's not possible for a mother to be attuned to her child 100 percent of the time, but even 20 to 30 percent of the time is sufficient to create a strong foundation in a girl's health and sense of self that will stay with her for the rest of her life. Hence the term "Good Enough Mother," for "good enough" will do just fine. However, if that minimum percentage isn't met, and the daughter's emotional needs are ignored often enough, then there are dire consequences. The daughter will become so overwhelmed by these unbearable feelings that over time they will become trauma — unmet, undigested emotional experiences that stay lodged in the subtle and physical bodies — that she may carry with her for her entire life. She'll constantly feels like she's falling or being "dropped." Once she realizes that there's no hope of being truly held by her mother (or perhaps even both parents), she loses trust in her mother, herself, and the world.

This crucial bonding that does (or does not) happen between a mother and her baby sets the stage for the rest of the child's life. For us as women, it influences how in touch we are with our gut feelings and even how prone we are to addiction. Recent studies show that addictive behavior may be linked to the poor development of oxytocin (the "love" hormone released during breastfeeding and mother-child bonding) in small children.[4] Exposure to stress and trauma before age three may impair the development of oxytocin and therefore make some people more likely to abuse drugs or alcohol. The success rate of bonding also influences how resilient we are in the face of stress and disease, how well we are able to self-regulate our needs and emotions, whether or not we view the world as safe and benevolent, and how well we connect with others.

If you did not grow up with all of the qualities of a loving holding environment (because, unfortunately, many of us didn't), it's necessary and welcome to grieve that. However, be sure not to stay in the anger and sadness for too long. Remember, our journeys start with psychological healing, but this step is only the beginning. Rather than pointing our fingers at our mothers, we need to grow up and give ourselves what they didn't. The Heroine's Journey is a path of taking strong responsibility for your life and therefore cannot progress unless you learn how to attune to *yourself.*

The Four-Part Check-In

This practice helps us to heal old beliefs that our feelings are bad and dangerous, our physical needs are shameful, our bodies will betray us, and we can't trust our intuition.

At the start of each day, like a mother getting a read on her child's mood and well-being in the morning, tune into your inner landscape. Do this by checking in with the four layers of your being — body, mind, feelings, and SHE — to see how they're doing and what they need from you in the day ahead. Slowing down each day to the pace of your feeling body allows the more subtle dimensions of your inner world to surface when they feel safe, allowing them to reveal to you the gifts within their hidden dimensions.

It's important to write this process down in your journal rather than merely thinking about it. The act of writing gives you much more clarity, and it takes only a few minutes.

1. Body: How is your body feeling today? Is a particular part calling for attention? What is it trying to tell you? Given all of this, what does your body need from you today?

2. Mind: This is often the easiest of the four parts to connect with since, for better or worse, we're often lost in thought. What are the main thoughts you're experiencing? What have you been thinking about for the past few hours? Few days? Is there a continual loop or fantasy you're playing or obsessing over? Given all of this, what does your mind need from you today?

3. Feelings: Here's where we have the least amount of awareness — and vocabulary. We live in a world that doesn't make space for our feelings. What are your dominant feelings today? Write down as many of them as you can. Don't worry if they're contradictory. They often are! What are these feelings trying to communicate to you? How can you give more support to your feelings today? What do they need? What are you *not* wanting to feel?

4. SHE: What is your intuition, feminine soul, or inner wise woman saying? What does SHE need you to do or know right now? What would bring you harmony and balance today? What would make you incredibly happy today? Whatever answer arises, the first thing that comes up — either as an inner voice or a flash of knowing — is your SHE speaking to you. The *second* thing that comes up is your mind responding (so listen to the former).

It's one thing to recognize your needs, and it's another one to actually *meet* those needs. Make it a top priority each day to meet the essential needs of these different layers of yourself. This approach will offer you a new paradigm for working with your needs and feelings, one that's *responsive* rather than neglectful or reactive. *This* is how you begin to mother yourself.

Attunement for Adults

One of my earliest memories dates back to preschool. Alone in the blue-tiled school bathroom, I sat on the toilet, feet dangling beneath me, my urine-drenched overalls crumpled around my ankles. I hadn't wanted to inconvenience anyone because I had to go to the bathroom, so I had held it, and held it, and held it — until I couldn't hold it any longer. This denial of my own needs continued in varying degrees into my adult years: working too long without taking a break, staying up too late even when I was tired, saying yes to invitations when I really wanted to stay cozy on the couch.

We're raised to be good girls, diminishing our own needs while prioritizing those of others. When our parents either shamed or didn't listen to our needs, we cut ourselves off from our inner guidance, creativity, free expression, and even our own unique likes and dislikes.

In what ways do you ignore your own needs? Do you neglect to drink water when you're thirsty? Do you eat things that you know don't make you feel well? Do you engage in relationships that make you feel lousy? If we all take an honest look, there are numerous ways on any given day that we abandon our innermost needs. Let's practice some self-care, right here and now. Ask yourself: How can I make myself 5 to 10 percent more comfortable right now? Pause and listen to the answer. Now follow through and do that before moving on. I'll wait!

Just as first-time parents have no idea what they're doing when they bring their infant home from the hospital, right now you might not have any idea how to begin attuning to yourself. That's okay. All that's needed is your willingness and your presence. Simply showing up is the first step.

Whether or not we have children, as women we can all relax into our neurology. We're hard-wired for motherhood. Deep down, we really *do* know how to do this! We know how to cultivate an inner holding environment where we're undistracted, available, and interested in what's arising internally. We know how to be curious about how we're feeling — physically, emotionally, mentally, and spiritually.

To begin, bring awareness to whatever's arising (a rumble in your belly, the heat of anger in your chest, or incessant worrying about the kid who's bullying your child at school). This brings you halfway to attunement, because awareness of what's arising is the "contact" piece. Next, allow whatever's arising to fully be present, without pushing it away (in the case of unpleasant stimuli) or craving more of it (with pleasant stimuli). This allows you to create "space."

Buddhism teaches us to cultivate the skill of attunement through the practice of mindfulness meditation. With an inner atmosphere of kind, all-pervading awareness, we acknowledge whatever arises within and around us. We allow this moment to be exactly as it is, without interference. Through this, something rather miraculous starts to happen: deep healing. Neuroscientists have yet to figure out exactly how this works, but through the simple act of intrapersonally meeting *ourselves* by acknowledging and giving space to what is, we allow obstacles to be digested and integrated. This process of splitting our own attention into the caregiver and the one who is cared for imitates the attunement between a mother and her child. As Buddhist psychiatrist Mark Epstein proposes, when we neither underreact nor overreact to our experiences, "The clear-eyed comprehension of suffering permits its release."[5]

For women who didn't grow up in empathic households, the first step to healing may be to seek out empathic relationships and environments: a therapist, meditation retreat, compassionate mentor, support group, or even a friend who listens well. In these safe spaces, over time the undigested trauma we've accumulated during and since our childhood will start to surface, and when it does, it's important to remember that this is an essential part of the process. Healing isn't about stopping pain. Usually we have to feel worse before we can feel better. The unpleasant feelings that surface within these loving containers hold the very medicine we need to heal.

Healing Your Childhood Trauma

There's no one point in your life when you'll be completely healed, because simply being alive is a traumatic experience. We're fragile beings, and every day we're reminded of this — whether it's because we missed a flight or had a fender bender. Little and large upheavals are an actuality in everyday life. Because of this frequently arduous randomness we all face each day, we can often feel like motherless daughters.

Tending to all layers of our inner worlds each and every day, and ideally multiple times throughout each day, builds our capacity to face life's unpredictable nature. When we develop this tool to work with our trauma, it becomes a doorway to our illumination. Each doorway then leads to another doorway in this ongoing process, and the path continually reveals new layers of ancient wounds as we go.

When you follow this path, for a stretch of time you feel relatively secure and settled, like you're "winning" at the game of life. Then you bump up against an obstacle. Things get shaken up, inside and out, and life knocks you to your knees again.

As you may have already experienced, this oscillation occurs at an even more accelerated rate during a long meditation retreat, because sitting still and putting aside our habitual thoughts for hours, days, and sometimes weeks on end prompts deeper feelings (not just the pleasant ones!) to bubble up from our depths. Yet it's during these transitory times that the Heroine's Journey escalates. During retreats we can heal things that might take decades to process in therapy, which is one of the many reasons why participating in retreats needs to be a regular part of every woman's life.

There's no way to predict how these traumas will surface for you. Undigested past experiences may emerge from your unconscious through your dreams, wordless feelings, spontaneous tears, or just a deep "je ne sais quoi" malaise. The best way to prepare yourself is through a daily mediation and self-attunement practice, and also by hearing stories from others. That way, when your own ancient grievances feel safe enough to air themselves, you'll be able to recognize what's arising and get the appropriate support.

Some of my childhood trauma, experienced as repressed rage, arose in me during the upheaval I recounted in the Introduction. It didn't seem connected to any particular person or incident, so I went to see my therapist, Diana, to help me work through it. Rather than toughing it out alone, whenever we know we're stretching into a new level of consciousness that we need support in navigating, it's time to reach out for help. When we can't hold our own inner ground, we need to find a skilled, empathic other to hold it for us. Here's an example of how Diana created an empathic holding environment for the bound-up energy inside me to organically release.

"Now, what brings you here today?" Diana probed as we sat facing one another, cross-legged on the floor.

"I feel like I'm going crazy," I blurted out.

"Mmm," she nodded, eyes full of compassion.

"I feel so stuck. I have so much energy inside my body right now. So much rage in my belly. I don't know what to do with it. I don't know what's happening to me."

"Okay, okay," she soothed. "Slow down. Put your hands on your belly and feel the energy there as you talk to me."

I nodded and followed her cue, sliding my hands across my belly, then down, feeling my legs.

"You've had to be such a good girl," she continued, "Soooo perfect. So controlled."

My lips began to quiver as tears flowed down my cheeks.

"Keep moving," she whispered, nodding to the physioball to her left.

I crawled over and rested my belly on top of it.

"Good," she encouraged.

Coming back to my tears, she added, "It's not your fault."

"What do you mean, *it's not my fault*?" I asked, incredulous.

"Oh, sweetie," she cooed, "you didn't do this to yourself. Your mother wanted you to be perfect in the way she never was, just as your grandmother tried so hard to make *her* perfect. Your mom didn't know any other way. It's no one's fault. Look, I know this can be hard to hear, Sara. I can stop at any time, just say the word."

Still looking down, I nodded for her to continue and kept rocking my belly over the ball.

"This is a moment *every* woman has to face in life if she wants to be a *conscious* woman. It's time for you to get your mother out of your cells," she said slowly.

I stopped moving, thinking about her words.

"Open your jaw and move it around. Let some sound out," she guided. "Whatever you do, don't freeze up. Okay?"

I nodded.

"Keep breathing, keep moving your hips a little bit, don't lock up. We don't need to do anything you don't want to do. We don't need to move too quickly. We can just go at your pace, okay?"

Moving to a place inside beyond words, I nodded again, my ponytail sweeping down against the sides of the rubber ball.

"You can scream right here, right now, if you want," she offered.

I looked up at her quizzically.

"Yes, you can do whatever you want here. And if you want to scream, you can just come off the ball and lie down right here."

Without thinking, my body followed her words, landing on the rug right in front of her lap.

"Yes, just like that, good."

I lay down on my back, bending my knees so my feet rested beneath them. *Don't do this*, an inner voice warned. *You'll make a fool out of yourself.* My body listened to Diana, not that old, familiar good girl voice.

"Good, keep moving, like you did on the ball. Like that, rocking your pelvis forward and back. Don't freeze up. Yes."

She paused, watching me closely.

"And don't just keep the movement in your pelvis; let it come all the way up to your head and your jaw. Don't leave them out of the flow. Right. Good. Now open your jaw, stretch your jaw. Stick your tongue out."

Everything about this feels awkward. I followed her voice. We kept going.

With closed eyes, I heard Diana release a loud grunt — one that made me think she did this often, unlike me.

"You try now."

And I did — mine coming more from my throat, hers coming more from the earth.

"Let's keep going like this together, okay?" she invited. "See if you can let go of your mind here. Just stay with the sound."

I've done this before. I know I have. Many times. I know how to do this. I do. I really do. It just takes one dive, and then I'll be there, on the other side of my fear, on the other side of what my mind has to say about all of this.

I curled my knees into my chest, and Diana placed one hand on each foot, asking me to PUSH my feet into her hands, like a laboring mother. Pushing, pushing, pushing: a roar exploded from my belly. The floorboards quaked. My mind was gone, so far gone that I forgot to even worry if anyone had heard me. My hands, bound into tight fists, beat the floor beside me — *dum, dum, DUM* — as I continued to roar.

My spine arched and I tilted my head back, freeing a low, deep wail all the way from the lips of my vagina to my throat.

Ten, fifteen, twenty minutes passed? I lost track of time. We stayed together like that until my cries faded into silence. Only soft tears and a soft belly remained.

"That was really good, Sara. Really, really good." Diana smiled. She was sitting next to me now like a watchful mother.

Opening my eyes, I saw her through my blur of tears, and I smiled back.

"I hope this wasn't too much for you. Are you okay?" she asked with concern.

I nodded my head. "Yes, I'm okay."

I rolled to my side and carefully came up to a sitting position.

"Look into the mirror," she suggested. "Look into your eyes. See yourself."

I turned from her to my own reflection in the mirror on the wall in front of us. My mascara was smeared all around my eyes, forming muddy black rivers down my cheeks. My hair had sprung out of my ponytail. I felt both awed and disgusted at what I saw; I looked ugly, raw, and unkempt.

"You look like a wild woman," Diana laughed, "because now you are!"

I partly laughed and cried. Yes, wildness, that's what I saw.

"You're so powerful, sweet Sara," she hushed behind me, not wanting to disturb this union with this new part of myself. "So, so powerful. So, so beautiful. So, so strong. Welcome home, Sara."

At some point along your journey, you too will need to release the rage you hold for your mother, in your own way.

The Divine Mother Enters through the Wound

My experience with Diana showed me that I didn't need to fix, change, or get rid of anything in order to heal. Being exactly where I was, within a loving holding environment, was all I needed to take me where I wanted to go. I just needed to feel safe in acknowledging and expressing what I had lived my whole life thinking was *un*lovable and *un*acceptable. I left her office that day knowing that my rage wasn't wrong. My perfectionism wasn't bad. My mother wasn't to blame. In fact, because I survived my childhood, to the point of being able to learn from my trauma, my mother and I both had done a "good enough" job. And that was more than enough. Also, at a deeper level, I started to understand that it was no coincidence these two seemingly disparate things arose together — the radical acceptance of such a messy part of my past, and the felt sense that the cosmic love of the Mother Goddess had been holding me all along.

We usually look for the Divine Mother in roses, rivers, and song. We never expect in a million years that we'll find Her in the very manure pile we're standing in, trying so desperately to escape. We're untrained at picking up Her polite knocks (*tap, tap, tap,* says our intuition!) at the front door of our fortresses. We don't answer. So SHE goes around to the rear, banging on the back door. SHE shakes up some havoc in our lives, trying with a bit more might to get our attention (*bang, bang, bang!*). Still, no luck. Finally, SHE enters the only way that SHE can, by slipping through an itty-bitty crack in a cellar window. SHE enters through the parts of us we've stopped abiding in long ago — the darkest, murkiest rooms of our inner homes that we didn't have the capacity to face as little girls. When we learn to mother ourselves well enough to bring these soul lesions in our cellars to the surface, they become the very portals through which SHE enters.

For this reason, the Divine Mother shines as the most venerated goddess in the world. Across all continents, devotees report apparitions of Her. Each tale speaks of divine healing, relentless mercy, and grace. On a yellow sticky note on the bulletin board above my computer, I scribbled the following:

Goddess = SHE who sweetens all things

Like a mother singing a lullaby to her sick baby in the wee hours of the night, the Mother Goddess can sweeten the inexplicable traumas we face throughout our lives. When we open to Her, the Mother heals all wounds through Her capacity to hold in perfect love even what we label as the lowliest parts of ourselves.

Ventilating the unhealed pain of our childhoods allows us to forgive ourselves and our mothers. This opens up space for us to understand what the "Mother" *really* is — true nourishment, incredible sweetness, and relentless mercy. The Heroine's Journey therefore begins in the wombs of our biological mothers, accelerates when we learn to be good mothers to ourselves, and ends with the remembrance that we're always perfectly held in the lap of the Divine Mother. We are all Her daughters. We're stronger when we're connected to Her. When we remember this, the Mother's love can pour into us so that we too can then be forces of unconditional love for the world. This very process is the Heroine's homecoming that we're moving so steadfastly toward.

Let's look now at the core feminine spiritual practices that will help take us there.

Journaling Questions

- Explore your relationship with your mother (or mother figure) right now. If she's not alive, recall what it was like before she died.
- What do you know about your mother's childhood? What was her relationship with your grandmother? Do you notice any similarities between the generations?
- What trauma from your past have you not fully recognized or digested because you feel ashamed or afraid of it?
- Have you ever experienced divine love? Think back to your childhood, or pivotal moments in your life when grace seemed to pervade an otherwise ordinary moment. Recall as much as you can about those experiences.

Chapter 4

Crafting a
SHE-Centered Life

How we live our days is how we live our lives.
— Annie Dillard, *Teaching a Stone to Talk*

A woman's spiritual life is an evolution. She must build it herself. Stepping onto the feminine spiritual path feels very much like wandering into a magical forest. There's no clearly paved road. The circumstances of our lives guide us. We find our way through trusting what we're drawn to. Rather than adhering to a prescribed dogma, we sculpt our path from the inside out, adapting lineages and heritages until we feel congruity between inner and outer, above and below. Looking back through the ages, we see that every spiritual leader who has made a lasting contribution to this world gathered her wisdom from a plethora of sources. She was able to do this because she was so rooted in herself that she didn't get lost or swept up in any one "right" way or point of view.

In my early twenties, I attended my first women's yoga class. An avid Ashtanga practitioner (or "Power Yogi") at the time, I felt very out of my element and shyly set up camp next to a sunny window in the back left corner of the yoga studio. Sitting down gingerly in the middle of my frayed, purple mat, I watched the teacher, Marilyn, as she closed the door to the hallway and sashayed over the creaky floorboards to her own mat in the front of the room. Although I had heard she was in her fifties, Marilyn seemed to be part sixteen-year old, part elder. She emanated an ineffable shine. *She doesn't look like all the other "accomplished" yoginis I know!* I thought to myself.

Neither tightly sculpted nor rail-thin, her flesh flowed like a roaring summer creek: wild, soft, powerful. Her belly, an unfamiliar mixture of round and toned, moved with her breath beneath her snug lavender tank top. A delicious contradiction, Marilyn scrambled everything I thought a "good spiritual practitioner" *should be*. Could one really be strong *and* soft? Whimsical *and* dedicated? That day, Marilyn blessed me with a humbling realization: I had inadvertently smuggled with me onto my spiritual path the exact pseudo-masculine ideals of power and success that I came to yoga and meditation to get away from! And it turned out that class with Marilyn was ceremonious in an even bigger way, because she was the person to first introduce me to her teacher, Sofia Diaz, thus initiating me on my path as a yogini.

As you read this chapter, notice your own desire for a neat and tidy map of what feminine spiritual practice is. I'm not going to give you that well-packaged plan. No one can give you this. You have to create your own. I *can* provide you with a set of principles that I find to reign in this vast, magical forest, and that you can use as your compass along your own yogini path. Keep in mind that even these principles cannot be set in stone. You, or another wise being in your world, might have some to add or delete; that's okay. As we're resurrecting the lost art of feminine spiritual practice, we'll need to be fluid and collaborative as we define it.

1. Cultivate a Daily Practice and Sacred Space

An inward-guided life only comes from ongoing practice. This takes time, discipline, and devotion. Daily rituals ground us, allowing all of our actions to align with our deepest priorities. Just like you can't win the Olympics without training every day, you can't become a Heroine without carving out time every day for *communing with* and *becoming* Her. We each need to create a strong container for our daily training times, for a daily practice of yoga, meditation, prayer, energy cultivation, and self-inquiry serves as the foundation of this work. If you don't already have an established daily practice and teacher, you can use my first book to learn more about my complete philosophy and approach to practice, as well as to obtain specific instructions for each of the components, or you can find an alternate source of instruction

Depending upon your level of experience and availability, carve out anywhere between ten minutes to three hours each day, first thing in the morning, to connect with yourself and the Sacred. What you do first thing each morning impacts how you experience the rest of the day. This is when you're most receptive and vulnerable, so make sure that the outer messages and agendas you're pursuing nourish and anchor you in your depths. Before you wear all of your other roles in life, put yourself in your own sacred space where you can relax all of your external masks and rest in your primordial nature. Take this commitment seriously. Daily practice is precious; it's what allows us to fully live during all the hours of the day.

Right when you wake up in the morning, rather than rolling over to check your phone, be intentional about your first thoughts. Make it a practice to fix your thoughts on your deepest dedication before getting out of bed. Recite to yourself a phrase, poem, or affirmation, and also consider your impermanence. Be grateful for a new day, and recognize that it could possibly be your last. How do you want to live it? Let your heart awareness marinate in these early contemplations for a few moments before even putting your feet on the ground. Then get up and, as soon as possible, enter your sacred space for your practice.

For this practice to take root in your life, it needs its own "holding environment." Create a sacred space in your home that's *just for you*. Keep this separate from your family, partner, and technology. Fill it with those things that most inspire you and remind you of your highest Self. This is the space where you'll connect with your SHE and your rich inner world. This is the space where you'll birth your new life and surrender all the outdated parts of yourself in the process. At another level, remember that this sacred space also lives within you, in your own body, your own inner home. Be sure to also find sacred spaces near where you live to seek refuge when you need to. Yoga studios can serve as modern-day temples, as can spaces in nature, meditation centers, and even quiet cafés that are off the beaten path.

2. Welcome Silence and Prayer

Silence is fast becoming an endangered species on this planet, and it's also your SHE's oxygen. Within silence, you open to divine communication: prayer. Prayer is a two-way conversation — offering and receiving — with your SHE. Aiming your thoughts toward Her, you ask for help, give thanks for your blessings, and listen for guidance and feedback about your next steps. The more silent you become, turning to Her for direction, the more SHE will communicate with you. Carve out time daily to commune with Her. Ask her to turn up the volume and to become a stronger, clearer presence in your life. Trust your experience. When you're engaged with Her, you're always given exactly what you need to grow.

3. Clarify Your Priorities

How can we possibly attain what we want if we don't even know what that is? We need to continually update our priorities to make sure we're going after the most meaningful things in life. In almost every interview I gave while on tour for *The Way of the Happy Woman*, the interviewer asked, "What's the one thing every woman every day can do that will have the biggest impact on her happiness?"

I always offered the same answer: "Sit in silent meditation for ten minutes a day."

We're *all* busy. But no matter how full you think your plate is, you can spare ten minutes. How do you do that? To start, recognize that you can't just start doing something new (like meditate for ten minutes a day). First, you have to stop doing something else (like surfing the Web in the morning). Back up and take the big view. In your journal, write down the top three priorities in your life, in their order of priority. Now look at your day today. How are these three priorities represented? Eliminate or reduce anything that isn't one of your top three priorities in order to find the time to live the life you want to live, daily.

4. Leave Open One Third of Your Space for SHE

You know how you get sick or injured when you're moving too quickly through life and have taken on too much? If you don't make space for your journey, that space will be thrust upon you. While the following recommendation is unconventional, it shows what's required for changing the status quo. Based on the present season of your life, adapt and interpret these guidelines in whatever way feels congruent with your current lifestyle needs.

Ancient healing sciences like India's Ayurveda teach us to always leave one third of our stomachs empty when we're eating a meal for optimum digestion. Any less than that leaves our bodies overwhelmed and unable to optimally extract the nutrients we need from our food. The same holds true for our inner worlds. What would it take for you to leave one third of the space in your calendar free for your SHE *each day*? If you're awake for fifteen hours a day, that's five hours of "being time." In one week that's about two and a half days. In one month that's about ten days. In one year that's about four months.

Your SHE space is your time to clear the decks of your usual responsibilities. It's a physical space and time dedicated to what feeds your soul. It's space where genius, inspiration, and healing can transpire. It's *being* time. When your SHE space dwindles and you spend all your time tending to your "outer world," exhaustion, self-doubt, disconnection, and a sense of being overwhelmed start to creep in.

If you want to live from your wisdom, joy, and depths, then you need to create the time and space to cultivate this. Plus, your SHE is shy. That's why the voice of intuition is always referred to as the "still, quiet voice within." When you're busy rushing around, engaging with other people all the time, there's no way that you can hear your SHE, much less live from Her.

On a single day, in your SHE space you could do your daily practice, write in your journal, go to a dance class, make art, hike in nature, visit with girlfriends, and/or sit on your porch and listen to the birds. This is space for you to fiercely guard those passions and pursuits that make you come alive. Every woman needs to protect her joy and her creative time. SHE space offers sustenance for your soul. Each month or season you could either go on a weekend retreat or have a stay-at-home retreat. Each year you could go away for a weeklong retreat to replenish your inner wellspring.

Take a Daily Digital Detox

Technology is quickly eating up all of our time. We're addicted to our devices, and no wonder: every time we check our email or social media we enjoy a dopamine surge in our brains. We now even experience that little high every time we simply glance at our phones. No wonder we can't stop looking at them, much less put them down and actually turn them off!

Here lives a *huge* opportunity to create more SHE space. A little dare: For the next month, turn your devices completely off at least one hour before you go to bed each night. Instead of bringing them into the bedroom, invest in an old-fashioned alarm clock. Don't turn your devices back on until after you've done your practice, gotten dressed, and eaten your breakfast the next morning. Then, for at least twenty-four hours each week, take a digital "Sabbath." Tell your friends, family, and colleagues that you'll be offline completely. Once a year, unplug for a longer stretch of time (at least seven to ten days) to stay completely away from screens.

---

5. Practice Sensual Presence

During a retreat with one of my teachers, I proudly reported to her that I meditated for one hour every day. Her response was not what I expected: "Wonderful! And what are you doing the other twenty-three?"

Her perspective reminded me that every moment of the day can be SHE space, *if* we allow it to be. When we're nursing the baby, driving on the freeway, and chopping the onions, we can be at home in our bodies and alive in our senses. Rather than getting lost in thoughts, we can fully inhabit our lives.

6. Think: This *and* That, Not This *or* That

Bring all of yourself to this journey. There is no part of you that's not welcome here. The further you go, the more you should feel like you're naked, removing layer upon layer of masks, armor, roles, and identities that shield you and keep you in a protective cocoon of old, limiting habits.

Radical inclusion, *not* binary thinking, pulses at the heart of feminine spiritual practice. Just as the color white contains every hue of the rainbow, our aim is to feel and contain *everything* at once, without closing to any of it. Society condones only select expressions of femininity — namely the good girl and the mother. Can we each embody every possible emanation of womanhood? The witch? Seductress? Bitch? Wild woman? Queen? Priestess? A quick way to know where we're closed is to notice if we mind taking the form of any of these expressions.

Every experience along this journey is part of the journey. Exclude nothing. Welcome everything as an invitation to go deeper, and remember that, while I'm recounting this journey through the pages of this book, the real journey is always unfolding within you and your daily life.

7. Put Relationships at the Center

We need rhythms of being alone and being together, but throughout we're held in an interconnected web. While we will all pass through the gates of initiation alone, we can't get there alone. This means we need to put relationships at the center of our journeys — with ourselves, friends, family, lovers, and the divine.

Within these relationships, we need circles of supportive, like-minded women who understand this path, and with whom we can share both our triumphs and our stuck points. We need sisters who can see what's possible for us, without getting caught in the mire of petty competition.

Notice any aversion you have to being supported by other women, and keep moving toward it anyway. The relationships you have with other women mirror your relationship to the feminine at-large. As you heal your ties with other women, the effects will reverberate out to strengthen all other aspects of this journey.

Note: To join our free virtual sisterhood for support during this journey and beyond, please visit www.TheBookofSHE.com/practices.

8. Stop Being a Victim

Take 100 percent responsibility for your life. There are no scapegoats here. No blaming. No shaming. Any and every time that you point your finger at someone else (e.g., they hurt me; he took my power; she made me angry), see that only one of your four fingers points at that person. Your other three fingers are pointing back at... YOU. It's time to wake up to all the ways in which you are hurting *yourself.* Everything "out there" is a mirror for what's happening "in here." Stop living in the past through incessant blaming and regret.

See your past as a gift, for it brought you here. Without the challenges you've faced, you would have no reason to cultivate such inner strength, resilience, and power. Let go of the old story. It's time to write a new one. When you take radical ownership of your life, you can finally begin to heal. You can't hold the self-identity of victim and heroine simultaneously. Which will you choose?

9. Ask Yourself: Are You in Love?

In any moment, whether you're on the meditation cushion or on hold during a call with your airline's not-so-great customer service, there's one question you can answer yourself to know whether or not you're engaged in feminine spiritual practice:

Am I in love?

If the answer is no, then identify what needs to shift within you, right now — in your body, in your breath, in where you're placing your energy and attention — in order for you to be able to answer yes to this question.

That shift from no to yes is the essence of feminine spiritual practice. When we ask ourselves if we're in love and answer yes, we land back in our feminine nature: open, receptive, and available to all of life. Write this question on the back of your hand, on a sticky note, with a whiteboard marker on your bathroom mirror. Ask yourself this question often, and each time the answer is no, open to the changes that will shift your response to yes.

10. Zig and Zag

The Buddha often taught through storytelling, and one of his most famous tales was of the formation of "the Middle Way." A lute player, who was feeling discouraged in his meditation practice, approached the Buddha for advice: "Should I maintain tight control over my mind during meditation or should I just let my thoughts flow?"

In response to this musician's inquiry, the Buddha asked, "Well, what happens when you tune your instrument too tightly?"

"The strings break," the musician answered.

"And what happens when you string it too loosely?"

"No sound comes out," the musician answered, "for the string that produces a tuneful sound is neither too tight nor too loose."

"That," said the Buddha, "is how to practice: not too tight and not too loose."

If we are too loose with ourselves, we won't practice, much less even bother exerting the effort to live a life beyond our superficial concerns and personalities. Conversely, if we are too tight with ourselves, we feel tense, rigid, and too contracted to experience much of anything. To stay the course for the long term, we must learn to experiment with creatively zigging (e.g., doing our practice, eating well, remaining mindful and grounded, etc.) and zagging (e.g., sleeping in one morning, trading our yoga class for a matinee, or enjoying some unstructured time in the evenings rather than signing up for another online course). The more fluidly we can dance with the inevitable oscillations of our bodies, moods, and lives, the more successful we'll be.

There's no set prescription for when to zig or zag. We need to take our own best guess in every moment by remaining childlike. In order to learn anything new, we must be willing to trade in our confidence for awkwardness. Let's be like toddlers, fumbling and wobbling around, yet loose, light, and playful. Let's not take ourselves too seriously.

Remember to laugh, play, and be kind to yourself. To lose your sense of humor is a grave thing indeed! Treat yourself as you would your own daughter who's just learning how to walk. As Zen master Suzuki Roshi wrote in *Zen Mind, Beginner's Mind*, "In the beginner's mind there are many possibilities, in the expert's there are few."[1]

11. Transform Obstacles into Opportunities

We're neither expecting immediate results here nor trying to transcend the pains of this world. The goal isn't to eradicate obstacles, because that's not even an option. Instead, when we learn to tap into our immense creative potential (as discussed further in chapter 8), we can turn obstacles into opportunities.

To do this, our daily rituals must include two things:

1. Practices of actuality, or meeting what's here
2. Practices of potentiality, or envisioning what's possible

We practice actuality through presence, attunement, and mindfulness. This allows us to meet obstacles head-on, rather than running from them or wishing they were otherwise. Working skillfully with actuality strengthens our trust that life never gives us anything that we can't handle. The exact circumstances we're facing hold the key to where we want to go and who we want to become.

To practice actuality, each day recite to yourself one or both of the following intentions:

- Today I will use adversity as my path. It's here anyway, so I might as well meet it.

- Whatever circumstances are arising, may they serve to awaken wisdom and love in my heart and mind.

Use one as your "first thought" if that feels right. Allow them both to help you to reframe as opportunities any obstacles you're currently facing.

When you allow things to be as they are, something loosens. A portal opens. Your immediate experience becomes rich and satisfying — even if it's riddled with obstacles. When you fully embrace each moment, you're inhabiting the center of your life. There, you always find exactly what you need within you to grow.

This is where potentiality comes in. As you remember with childlike wonder how to activate your dusty, underused imagination, you envision what you most long for. What would make you incredibly happy? Who would you be and how would you feel if you were in vibrant, radiant health? What does your ideal day — and life — look and feel like? Take time each day to visualize and experience bodily, with all of your senses alive and engaged, what you most long for. We'll explore this more in chapter 12.

12. Follow the Signs

Feminine wisdom has gone underground, so we need to look to the Goddess in less obvious places, following underlying signs. SHE speaks through our dreams, recurring symbols and themes, and animal totems. SHE's everywhere, infusing our days with playful synchronicity. Willing to engage with anyone who's ready to pick up Her signal, SHE's constantly communicating with us.

What are the hidden messages coming up from Her through your unconscious, trying to make their way into the light of day? Are you listening? Do you know how to listen? In the daily rituals, silence and prayer, and SHE space discussed earlier in the first three steps, you can cultivate an inner and outer environment to speak with Her. Keep a dream journal. During your morning meditation, ask Her questions. Listen to Her answers. Learn how SHE speaks to you. Is it through words? A feeling in your body? Signs and synchronicity around you? Images in your mind? A combination of all of these?

13. Understand Feminine Wisdom: Change, Chaos, Cycles, and Spirals

Change

Impermanence is the bedrock of life. Everything is always in flux. We're always in transition. There's no end to change, and our bodies teach us this every day. Yesterday we were bloated; today we feel lean and sexy. Five minutes ago we felt excited; now we feel bored. Despite our obviously ever-changing realities, we all resist and fear change. *A lot.*

Take your seat in the part of yourself that is always here, that has never changed, and that will never cease to be. From that perspective, experience the poignancy of life's plethora of textures. Partake fully in the seasons of the year, and of your life. Rather than building your inner home upon a false ideal of stasis, learn to live in the fundamentally transitory, chaotic nature of existence. Balance comes not from remaining the same, but from maintaining flexibility in the midst of constant change.

Chaos

Chaos is the organizing principle of the universe. The Divine Feminine *is* chaos. The creative process *is* chaotic. Feminine wisdom reigns in the messy portals between destruction and creation, death and rebirth. SHE is the earthquake and the tsunami, and can neither be bargained or reasoned with. It's time to train yourself to trust and navigate from the very chaotic uncertainty that is your feminine nature. When things feel out of control, SHE is calling you home to a place of a more aligned, intrinsic order. Stay with the mess until that underlying order reveals itself to you. It will be far more magnificent than anything you could have concocted on your own.

Cycles

When we dive into the chaos, we discover an underlying rhythm and predictability. We start to hear the heartbeat of feminine wisdom alive and well within cycles. Women's moods and energy levels wax and wane like the moon, ebb and flow like the tides, flourish and decay like the seasons. Living in harmony with these cycles strengthens us, makes us wiser, and heals us. Denying them weakens our spirits, our bodies, and our connection to life herself.

Cycles help orient us when there are no external signposts in sight. How many times do we find ourselves in a rough patch and think, "Is this ever going to end? Will I ever be normal again?" Life's a constant rhythmic dance between dark and light. Remembering this helps us to acknowledge that we're far more resilient than we think we are. When we trust our cycles we know this: if our lives are falling apart, they will soon come back together again. We'll explore cycles more in chapters 7 and 8.

Spirals

The labyrinth represents our spiraling spiritual pilgrimage. Built into a labyrinth is inherent chaos. It has many twists and turns that sometimes seem to lead us further away from our goal, yet they always miraculously land us right smack in the center of it. Once we find ourselves in the middle, we think it's the end, but we're only halfway there!

Labyrinths can be confusing, but not impossible, to traverse, so long as we stay focused, present, and centered in ourselves. No two people walk the labyrinth in the same way, and each time we walk one, like snakes, we shed another skin and come closer to our core essence.

The Triple Goddess: Maiden, Mother, Crone

Here's a powerful archetype of feminine wisdom that holds each of these qualities: change, chaos, cycles, and spirals. In neopaganism, the Triple Moon Goddesses symbolize the circular web of life and rebirth. A version of the holy trinity, each represents a stage in a woman's life — Maiden, Mother, Crone — as well as the lunar cycle. When a woman passes through each of these three stages, she arrives in mature, empowered feminine wisdom — regardless of her age. During different phases of our lives, one dimension of this archetype will be more active than the others. Part of knowing and participating in our dynamic power is being able to access any one of these three at will.

The Maiden: She represents the spring, dawn, waxing moon, birth, puberty, beginnings, and eternal youth. She's coy, enchanting, carefree, independent, graceful, and innocent. She is open to new experiences and unafraid of the unknown. She knows how to play, dance, and embrace the child within.

The Mother: The heart of the Great Goddess, she represents the summer, midafternoon, full moon, marriage, parenthood, knowledge, increased confidence, and the culmination of an idea, desire, feeling, or relationship. More natural for most of us to relate to, she's the nurturer, teacher, and counselor who sustains and gives life. She is the keeper of seasons and cycles, holding wisdom in her core. She teaches by example. Her womb is the cauldron for creating a new baby, habit, relationship, or project. All of her creations are sustained by unconditional love, yet not without patience and discipline. Because the Mother is in touch with her personal responsibility and the consequences of all of her actions, the cultivation of the Crone begins during this phase.

The Crone: The Crone is the most misunderstood in this triad, for the more we fear death, aging, and the unknown, the more we fear this aspect of ourselves, and this stage of our lives. The witch, dark mother, hag, or silver-haired wise one, she represents winter, nighttime, menopause, the waning and dark moons, death, endings, transitions, and shadow work. Deep in her bones, she holds hard-earned wisdom, cultivated over a lifetime. The Crone uses her head — no longer just her emotions — to rule her choices. When you're at a crossroads in life, she's the one to go to, for she'll give you the most reliable feedback. Marion Woodman teaches that the root of the word *crone* is *crown*, and if a woman has done her inner work prior to this point, it is she who guards the treasures of the underworld, serving as a healer to her family, community, and the world.[2] Any woman who wants to experience the power of her wholeness must undergo her initiation into a Crone. We'll explore the Crone more in chapter 8.

14. Embody the Radiance Principle

As women we're born to shine. We're drawn to sequins, sparkling jewelry, and body glitter for a very good reason: we *are* embodied light. To live as a goddess incarnate, acknowledge, activate, and enhance your radiance daily. Hatha yoga (or the physical practices of yoga) open and illuminate the lines of light, or *nadis*, in our bodies. Cleansing ourselves of toxins allows us to shed cloaks of dullness. Honoring the potent medicine of beauty calls out to the splendor and light within. Buy flowers for your home. Light candles. Take time to keep your living space clean and lovely. Nurture and care for your body, as she is. Then stretch out of your comfort zone and take on the art of sacred adornment in ways that feel authentic to you: paint your nails, wear flattering clothes, do your hair and makeup. Cultivate and celebrate the divinity of your embodiment. We'll explore this more in chapter 10.

15. Include Your Sacred Anatomy

Your real feminine power lives "down there" — in your ovaries, uterus, and yoni (the Sanskrit word for "vagina," which I prefer to use over vagina, not as a euphemism, but because it points to both its physical and divine nature). Within our pelvises live our temples of transformation, and our yonis are the gateways between our inner creations and the outer worlds.

Even if any or all of these sacred creative organs have been removed, they still maintain a strong, energetic presence in your body that you can draw upon. Unless you include your reproductive organs in your yoga and meditation practices — and in all that you create in your life — you will never be able to make magic, know and express your feminine power, or express the radiance that is your true feminine nature. We'll explore this more in chapter 7.

16. Stay at Your Honest Edge

There's no such thing as halfway there. There are no shortcuts. Real yoga — union — transpires when you meet your honest edge and learn to cherish your greatest challenges. What yoga poses do you abhor? What feelings can you simply not bear to feel? Where in your life do you collapse, explode, or run away? Answer those questions for yourself, for that's where the gold lives. Whatever you're most afraid of is exactly the place where you need to grow next. You need mini-doses of going to your edge every day (staying for three minutes in a squat pose on your yoga mat, or sitting motionless in meditation while a fly crawls on your cheek) in order to train yourself to *stay* during the larger edges you face during a life crisis. We'll explore this more in chapters 8 and 11.

17. Live: Thy Will Be Done

Hand it all over to Her. Surrender. Radically trust that SHE has your back. SHE's holding you through all of this. Yes, SHE does move in mysterious ways. SHE's wily and playful and has a wicked sense of humor. SHE's pulling all the strings, but only in service of your truest, deepest, most embodied feminine realization. SHE wants you to win, and SHE's going to create the exact circumstance, in your life and in your own body, that you need to reign. Your practice, your every thought and life circumstance, even your reading this book right now is not random! Trust that SHE's guiding you, through all of this.

Find a picture that represents Her. SHE can be an archetype like Mother Mary, Tara, Kwan Yin, Aphrodite, or Lakshmi. SHE could be an image of nature, like the ocean or a tree. Place Her on your altar in your sacred space. Each day, physically bow to Her. See yourself laying all of your dreams, problems, and questions at Her feet. Let everything go, as an offering to Her.

Opening Ritual: Meeting Your SHE

I recommend gathering now the following supplies for our journey:

- A journal, used exclusively for this process.
- A special candle for your altar to light each day that you're on this journey.

- A daily offering for Her. This should be something from the natural world — a fresh flower, leaf, seashell, piece of fruit or incense, and so forth — to place on your altar each day. After twenty-four hours, bring this outside and give it to the earth. If it's edible, eat it. This represents your knowing that SHE is alive and inviting Her presence more fully into your life.
- A dedicated sacred space that can grow strong and rich with Her presence to hold the entire arc of your transformation.

Let's gather to commence our journey. See yourself crossing the threshold from your "normal" life into this liminal space. Sense all the women who are now taking their own Heroine's Journey joining together in a sacred circle. Know that we are all in this together. At no point along this pilgrimage have you ever been, or will you ever be, alone.

Look around the circle and find your seat. What does it look like? Sense its color, dimensions, shape, and style. Once you find the one that's destined to be your one-and-only Heroine's throne, sit down. Take your seat, sister.

From your seat, close your eyes, and listen deep inside. Hear your deepest intention. It's something to unearth, not something to contrive.

- What brought you to this journey?
- What do you most long to give, receive, and experience by taking this pilgrimage?

Take some time now to write down your intention in your journal. Write your intention in the first person and present tense, beginning "I intend to." If you wish, you can share this in our online SHE Circle.

When you feel complete, please come into a comfortable, meditative posture, with your spine long, and begin the visualization below.

To listen to the following visualization, go to www.TheBookofSHE.com /practices, to download the audio file. I've also included it in written form here. It's important that you actively engage your imagination by listening to this, and to all future visualizations in this book. If you only read these, you're merely using your rational mind and not drawing upon the deeper powers of your subconscious mind.

Take five slow, deep, and even breaths, inhaling for a count of five and exhaling for a count of five. Let your mind follow each breath. Inhale into any physical tension you feel. Exhale, release it. Inhale into any pre-occupying emotions. Exhale, release them. Inhale into any thoughts or dominant mind forms. Exhale, release them. Inhale into any sounds or distractions in the room. Exhale, release them. Inhale into your whole body; exhale, release.

Next, get in touch with your earthing cord (from chapter 2). Feel a thick cord extending from your belly down into the center of the earth. Clearly envision each end of the cord. Inhale earth energy up through the cord and your legs. Exhale; circulate it in your body to any place that needs it. If at any time you start to feel distracted or overwhelmed during this visualization, reestablish this earth connection.

Now imagine that your torso is your inner home. See what this home looks like from outside. Is it a mansion? A hut on the beach? A tree house? See exactly what your home looks like. Notice what color it is and the materials it's made out of.

Once the details come into view, walk up the pathway toward the house. See what the front door looks like. Open it, cross the threshold, and step into the entryway. What does the inside of your home look like? What does it feel like? Walk through and explore the house until you find your sacred space, your personal temple. Peek around corners and into rooms. Or perhaps you already know exactly where your inner temple is.

See if there's a special door or hallway you need to pass through in order to enter your temple. Before you do, remove your clothes and shoes. See a place to bathe in fresh, clean water. Step in and dive under-water, feeling any dimensions of your old life that you're ready to release now washing away.

When you feel complete, see yourself stepping out of the water and drying yourself off. There's some clean clothing waiting for you. Put that on and notice what it is — a special outfit for your initiation. Dress slowly and ceremoniously, taking as much time as you need to.

When you're ready, walk through the doorway into your inner tem-ple. Once inside, look around. Notice everything you see — the walls, the floor, the smells and decorations. Perhaps it's a space outside in nature. Take some time to walk through it, exploring it more, taking it all in.

Now, walk over to the temple's altar. What kinds of adornments fill the altar? What images, flowers, candles, offerings?

Look down into your hands and see that you hold a special gift to place on your temple's altar as an offering for your journey. See what that is, kneel down, and place it on the altar. Say any prayer or blessing that feels right for you.

When you feel complete, take your seat in the temple, wherever you feel most comfortable.

Across the room, see a golden, shimmering light. From within this emerges the most beautiful, luminous goddess you've ever known. This is your SHE. Slowly, SHE walks toward you. What do you see? Try to sense and see everything about Her. What does SHE look like? Smell like? How does SHE make you feel? What is SHE wearing? What's the look on Her face and in Her eyes? What about Her hair? Look more closely. What's something about Her that you didn't see before?

Now, step a little closer and say hello in whatever way feels right. Ask Her if SHE has anything SHE needs to tell you. Pause and listen. SHE might speak in words, sounds, movement, symbols, or just a feeling you get from being with Her. If you need more time, pause until you feel complete with this step.

Receive what SHE has to say, and also take some time to ask Her any other questions you have for Her. When you feel complete, say goodbye in whatever way feels right.

When you're ready, say goodbye to this inner temple, and leave it the same way you came in. Know that you can return here at any time along your journey for inspiration, comfort, and connection with your SHE. SHE lives within you, always.

Once you've exited, walk back to the entryway of your inner home. Take some full belly breaths and slowly open your eyes.

Write down in your journal what you received from your meeting with your SHE. Write for at least ten minutes without stopping. Keep your pen moving with the stream of your consciousness, describing everything you can remember about your time down in your inner temple.

Please send out a prayer for all of our sisters as we begin our journey and resolve to travel this path for the benefit of all. And now, my dear sisters, we're as ready in this moment as we'll ever be. I'm holding the light. Let's go down.

Journaling Questions

- Which of these elements of a SHE-centered life do you feel you've already integrated into your life? Which ones do you feel inspired to integrate now?
- What obstacles do you perceive you will face in doing so? What support, inner and outer, can you draw on when you do?
- In what ways did your SHE feel familiar to you when you met Her? How did SHE surprise you?

Part II

The Descent

No tree, it is said,
can grow to heaven
unless its roots reach down to hell.

— Carl Jung, *Aion*

Emily Dickinson

Mount Madonna Retreat Center, Watsonville, California; May 2007

I wiggled to the edge of my cushion to sit up straighter. *God, I feel like she can see everything I'm feeling and thinking right now*, I moaned to myself. I drew in a few deeper breaths to try to smooth over my nerves. No such luck.

It was the first night of our five-day women's retreat, and she was half-way around the opening circle. Five more women until my turn. *Ba boom, ba boom, ba boom. Shhh,* I said to my heart.

Her wide brown eyes honed in like lasers on each woman as my peers "checked in" and shared their intentions for being there. Then Sofia gave each woman a name. Not her real name, but a name that came to her in that moment of introduction. A name that held, like a talisman, a truth for each woman to uncover during her time there on retreat. And, as would be my case, sometimes for much, much longer.

I don't remember what I said during my check-in that evening, but I do remember what came after that. A long, pregnant pause and then:

"I know! Your name is…Emily Dickinson!" Sofia squealed with a smile, her cheerful voice laced with a twinge of mischief.

Feeling slighted that I didn't get a more interesting or exotic name like "Tonga" or "Plumeria" as some of my peers had, I smiled demurely, then forced out a fake laugh in hopes that she would move on. I was growing increasingly uncomfortable with so many eyes on me.

A melancholic female poet. That's what I knew of Emily Dickinson. To this day, Sofia and I still laugh about how it was one of the most accurate and fated names that she has ever given anyone. My girlfriends who were on that retreat still call me Emily from time to time.

Seven years later, as I settled in to write this book, I met Emily again — not as a nickname, but as a leading lady in our Heroine's Journey. Emily Dickinson, indeed.

Chapter 5

Dancing with the Dark Goddess

One does not become enlightened by imagining figures of light,
but by making the darkness conscious.... Until you make the
unconscious conscious, it will direct your life and you will call it fate.

— Carl Jung , *Collected Works of C. G. Jung, Vol. 13: Alchemical Studies*

Can you guess what you, me, and Emily Dickinson *really* have in common? I found out last autumn when I drove to a cabin in Gold Hill, a mountain town twenty minutes up a windy road from Boulder, for a weeklong writing retreat. Holding in my heart the intentions to rest, replenish, and deeply connect with my SHE and the soul of this book, I put aside my usual retreat schedule and surrendered to synchronicity, opting to follow signs and intuitive nudges into the heart of my creative process.

In the mornings I mined old spiral-bound journals from as far back as my college years. I took copious notes on rehashed conversations, dreams, and insights from all the retreats I'd attended since then. I returned to scribbles and underlines that filled the margins in the mountain of books I had read on women's spirituality. One evening after dinner I cruised around the website of Sounds True, a local publishing company that features many of today's spiritual leaders. I was specifically looking for an inspiring audio talk to stream as I wound down from the day. As I searched its archives for Jungian analyst Marion Woodman, who offers fascinating insights into conscious femininity and addiction, I saw all the talks I'd already listened to.

Then: *Whoa. Wait. What's this?* One I hadn't seen before: "Emily Dickinson and the Demon Lover."[1] Without pausing to think, I purchased and downloaded it. For the next couple of hours, until well past my usual bedtime, I lay on the floor, looking out into the silent darkness, listening to Marion's earthy, passionate voice read Emily's poetry. Marion revealed a perspective into Emily's life that I'd never before heard. As proof of the canny wisdom of the Divine Mother in action, the more I listened to that audio, the more I knew She held a plan for this book far greater than what I could ever conceive of alone. Through this synchronicity, I felt She had just handed me a golden key. My doppelgänger, Ms. Dickinson, I learned that night, wasn't just a reclusive poet. She underwent the very transformation that we're undergoing here now. Her life's work, which arose out of deep heartache and introspection, proves how possible it is for *every* woman to transform her neurosis into her genius.

This alchemy can only transpire in our own inner, unconscious terrains. To continue on our journeys, it's time to explore the dark caverns of our bodies, souls, and psyches. Almost all cultures share a mythological theme that involves protagonists who are hurled into the underworld to face their fear of the darkness. Let's descend now into this underworld, step by step. Easy does it. Slowly now. We must first allow our eyes to adjust to the dark.

Two Kinds of Darkness

As a little girl, were you afraid of the dark? I used to envision green, googly-eyed monsters lurking under my bed, or slimy dragons slumbering in the lumpy shadows of my closet. We all grew up associating the dark with gloom and danger, even though it serves as the backdrop for our *entire* lives. As Clark Strand, author of *Waking Up to the Dark: Ancient Wisdom for a Sleepless Age*, notes, "Our lives begin in the womb and end in the tomb. It's dark on either side."[2]

We spend one third of our lives sleeping. For much of the year, darkness shrouds half of each day. Our lives are composed of interweaving, interdependent threads of light and dark. And still, darkness gets a bad rap. We're afraid of it. We resist it. We project it onto others. We avoid it at all costs. And for good reason. Darkness reminds us of our vulnerability. Slipping into night requires a surrender into deep, dreamless consciousness that most of us resist. We don't want to unplug, power down, and let go of "doing." We don't want to veer out of the capable, wakeful part of our being that we rely on so strongly to get by in life.

In fact, we're so frequently going, going, going that we've forgotten how to rest. We feel compelled to reach for the booze, the pill, the smoke, the secret late-night snack to help us check out. When we can no longer find the off switch, we have nightmares while still awake. We can't get off the freight train of our own minds.

Our demons stir at nighttime, or during the "dark nights of the soul." About 10 percent of Americans have chronic insomnia,[3] and many people — women especially — associate bed with trauma. Historically, people huddled together by candlelight or firelight at night to stay warm and protect each other. Now, most of us face our dark demons alone.

In fact, most of humanity has simply forgotten how to relate to darkness. Over the years, with the convenience of electricity, we've all become increasingly reliant on light. It allows us to be more machine-like, more productive. We can get things done at any hour. But is this really so wonderful? Probably not.

First, women's menstrual and hormonal cycles have been affected by this shift. Most of us no longer bleed with the cycles of the moon, since we're constantly exposed to artificial light. As well, we are all becoming increasingly disconnected from our intrinsic circadian rhythms, which affect appetite, the secretion of hormones, body temperature, alertness, and sleep timing. We're living in a time of darkness deprivation. Seen from outer space, our planet, plundered by light pollution, glows. Most of this nighttime light is completely unnecessary — streetlamps and shop lights staying on, even in unpopulated areas, through the wee hours of the night.

In order to heal, we need to remember how to value the night. We need to honor that this darkness is intelligent and necessary for our survival.

We can persist for weeks without food or water, but no one can live without sleep. We need to see the darkness as part of our nature. It's half of the miracle of life — a safe and holy place — imbued, like dark chocolate, with bittersweet beauty. We need to remember that all true creativity springs from the darkness. We need to learn to hold sleep, surrender, and uncertainty as profound spiritual practices.

At the same time, it's important to remember that not all darkness should be prized and cultivated. Just like Eskimos have many different words to describe snow, we too must become connoisseurs, discerning different breeds of darkness. While we want to adopt the fertile, pregnant darkness that represents the secret void, the spring soil, or cosmic womb that gives birth to all things (the *daemon*), we want to remain alert to the blackness of blindness and ignorance (the *demon*). The latter is a sleepy darkness, where we're plagued with the temptation to avoid facing our deepest truths.

In fact, if we can't face what the darkness is trying to teach us, the wisdom of the fertile void turns into evasion, and we choose to stay asleep, unresponsive to our call to grow. Rather, when we wish to heal ourselves, our aim is to be like Sumerian goddess Inanna, who gathered up the lost pieces of herself in the underworld. Unless we too are willing to collect the forgotten wisdom lost in the dark corners of our psyches, we'll experience resistance, rage, depression, illness, and addictions.

Demons and Daemons

If you bring forth that which is within you then that which is
within you will be your salvation. If you do not bring forth that
which is within you then that which is within you will destroy you.

— Elaine Pagels, *The Gnostic Gospel*

In my late teens and early twenties I found solace in odd places — with the great dames of literature who lingered dangerously on the dark side. I read Sylvia Plath's *The Bell Jar* three times and maniacally scoured her poetry and journals. I adapted Virginia Woolf's adage that every woman needs a room of her own. I adored Susanna Kaysen's bestselling memoir *Girl, Interrupted* and, even more so, Winona Ryder and Angelina Jolie's portrayal of this on the big screen. In retrospect, these women mesmerized me because a piece of their dazzling insanity also lived within me. My own paternal grandmother, Leona, whom I never had the chance to meet, suffered from bipolar disorder in a time before it could be diagnosed as such.

Each of these brilliant women didn't *quite* fit in. Infused with a spark of genius and fragile ego structures (or "holding environments"), they couldn't secure a place for themselves in a society that prized "normalcy" and conventional women, so they were banished into the borderlands of psychotic breakdowns. Constantly crisscrossing the paper-thin wall between brilliance and lunacy — without proper inner or outer support — none of these women fared well in the end. Sylvia committed suicide by sticking her head in an oven. Virginia suffered from bipolar disorder and drowned herself at the age of fifty-nine. Susanna ended up in a mental hospital. Leona smashed all the windows in my father's childhood home with a hammer, underwent electric shock therapy, and slit her wrists with a razor blade — although she did survive this attempt to end her own life.

Emily Dickinson also hovered all too near the centripetal lure of madness. However, in the end she was able to die a heroine rather than a victim. Like us, she was a "Father's Daughter," obsessed with meeting her father's standards of perfection in the presence of a mother who was both psychologically and emotionally absent. As a result, she sought masculine models of success and split her secret, inner world off from her outer world. Later in life, when she was no longer under her father's supervision, she projected her father onto another man and fell so deeply in love with him that she completely lost herself. When he eventually abandoned her, she had no inner resources to draw upon to cope with her grief. Completely devastated, she was almost suicidal.

Yet through her own sheer will and divine spirit, Emily prevailed. Rather than giving her feminine soul completely over to suicide, she sought another path and immersed herself in her own solitude. There, she began a daily writing practice — writing one poem a day for an entire year. It was those poems that made her famous, because in the depths she journeyed to within, Emily finally found her creative roots and her mature, feminine voice. Quite simply: her writing saved her life. She trusted her genius more than her brokenness, and in so doing, she successfully rewired her dark, destructive energy into artistic genius and psychological wholeness. Emily transformed her destructive darkness, or *demon*, into her fertile darkness, or *daemon*, thus embodying her soul's full, creative splendor.[4]

In his book *Grace and Grit*, the philosopher Ken Wilber explains this concept of *daemon* more fully.

> [*Daemon*] — the Greek word that in classical mythology refers to "a god within," one's inner deity or guiding spirit...[is] also known as...the tutelary deity or genius of a person, one's daemon...is also said to be synonymous with one's fate or fortune....[And] her own higher Self.[5]

Wilber elaborates that, as we saw with Emily, our demons and daemons are, ultimately, the same thing. Which direction they turn — into death or life — is entirely up to us. He continues:

> [There] is a strange and horrible thing about one's daemon. When honored and acted upon, it is indeed one's guiding spirit; those who bear a god within bring genius to their work. When, however one's daemon is heard but unheeded, it is said that the daemon becomes a demon, or evil spirit — divine energy and talent denigrates to self-destructive activity. The Christian mystics, for example, say that the flames of Hell are but God's love denied, angels reduced to demons.[6]

Just as the indigenous plants that grow directly around us hold the medicine for our ailments, the weeds of our inner demons contain the salve of our highest selves, or our SHEs. Rather than going to war with our demons or denying them by always striving for the "light," let's acknowledge that we cannot fully know our true, ecstatic nature as women without tapping into our dark sides. Have you grown tired of desiring one half of life, and always running from the other half of it? What if your true feminine power was waiting in that other half of life — the one you've been sedating, hiding, or hating?

Pain Is the New Pleasure; Ugly Is the New Beautiful

Approach that which you find repulsive!...
Anything you are attached to, let it go!...
Go to the places that scare you!

— Dampa Sangye to Machig Labdrön,
in Tsultrim Allione, *Feeding Your Demons*

The Buddha taught that our fundamental obstacle to true happiness resides in our incessant clinging to the eight worldly dharmas. We're always enmeshed in pursuing one or detesting the other. These include:

gain and loss
praise and blame
fame and disrepute
pain and pleasure

Round and round we all ride on the Ferris wheel of life. Sometimes we're up and sometimes we're down. No one can stay up forever. If this is a fundamental life truth, then why do we punish ourselves by always trying to make it otherwise? Only by finding equanimity, that part of ourselves that can hold steady through the entire Ferris wheel ride, regardless of where we are in the spectrum of "up" and "down," can we know true freedom.

Let's explore how these dualities operate in your own life. The outcome of this exercise will help you to clarify your personal demon/daemon dynamic and rest in the sweet spot between them.

Exploring Dualities

1. Fold a piece of paper in half, lengthwise.
2. On the left side of the paper, make a list of all the parts of yourself that you hate — body parts, relational tendencies, moods, and/or habits. From which of your behaviors do you suffer most? Think about the criticism from other people that stings you the most and that points toward a part of yourself that you also viciously judge. We'll consider these to be aspects of your "demon."
3. On the right side of the paper, next to each loathed aspect, write its counterpart. What's the opposing body part, expression, or activity that allows one of your hidden gifts to shine? What aspects of yourself deeply nourish you and those around you? Consider here what others praise you for most frequently. We'll consider these dimensions of your "daemon."
4. Look over both lists, side by side, seeing visually how they're two halves of a larger whole.

Here are some examples that some women in the SHE School unearthed:

Fat stomach — Strong Earth	Procrastinating — Creative
Tight — Juicy	Slutty — Sexy
Ungrounded — Connected	Controlling — Organized
Exhausted — Radiant	Martyr — Loving
Stuck — Curious	Grief stricken — Openhearted
Helpless — Powerful	Critical — Discerning
Judging — Appreciating	Intense — Passionate
Fear — Surrender	Raging — Fierce
Bossy — Powerful	Flat chest — Feminine nourishment

Let's take this even deeper. I first learned a version of the following meditation while on retreat with one of my teachers, the author and founder of Insight Yoga, Sarah Powers.[7] I frequently include this meditation in my morning practice because it helps me start my day with a felt sense of accepting my light and dark sides.

A Meditation for Embracing Your Opposites

Come to a comfortable, seated position, either on a chair with your feet flat on the floor, or cross-legged on a cushion. Make sure your hips are higher than your knees. Lengthen your spine, close your eyes, and place your palms facedown on your thighs. Drop your awareness down into your belly center. Take several natural breaths, concentrating on the sensations of your inhalation and exhalation.

Now, on your inhalation, recite internally, "I am willing to embrace my _____." (Fill in the blank with a "dark" quality from your demon list.) On your exhale, declare, "I am willing to embrace my _____." (Fill in the blank with the accompanying "light" quality from your daemon list.) Continue several rounds of this, using different opposing qualities for each breath cycle. You can also recite the eight worldly dharmas from page 105. Here are a few examples that I often use in my own practice.

Inhale: "I am willing to embrace my fear."
Exhale: "I am willing to embrace my courage."

Inhale: "I am willing to embrace my laziness."
Exhale: "I am willing to embrace my ardor."

Inhale: "I am willing to embrace my tiredness."
Exhale: "I am willing to embrace my vitality."

Inhale: "I am willing to embrace my failures."
Exhale: "I am willing to embrace my successes."

To complete, rest your attention back in your belly center for several breaths. Slowly open your eyes.

Advanced version: For experienced yoginis who already include alternate nostril breathing (or *nadi shodana*) in their daily practices, employ these recitations while using that breathing technique. Use one phrase on the inhale through one nostril and the opposing phrase on the exhale through the other nostril.

The Dark Goddess

In *Conscious Femininity*, Marion Woodman teaches that "The dark side of the feminine is vicious; it's a killer."[8] Learning how to listen to, love, and to integrate this fierce medicine is one of the most powerful gifts and daunting duties we have as women. She's Kali, Medusa, Pele, the Black Madonna, the witch who lives in the woods, or the dark woman who haunts the edges of your dreams. The fallen angel, plummeted from grace, She lives in the lower half of your body — in your anger, grief, loveless lust, and shame. She's not afraid of death, for She's the one who destroys. Her home is the cosmic void, the blackness of the womb before new life enters. The Dark Feminine stays coiled like a sleeping snake in your pelvis, waiting to either destroy or uplift you through your own repressed life force. She's the demon and the daemon, both.

One Saturday night, not long after my fiancé, Keith, and I first started dating, I commenced a more intimate dance with the Dark Feminine. That evening, which we were supposed to spend at Keith's house, I was besieged by a rough round of PMS that was even further amplified by the stress of sharing my first book with the world. I felt incredibly sensitive. Quivering inside, on the brink of breaking through my composed persona, my Dark Feminine started flowing strongly through me.

She was intense and unapologetic. Fiery and demanding. Angry and unreasonable. Lashing out and then turning back around and slapping me with criticism for doing so. She was completely overpowering my normal sense of "me."

I decided I wanted to go to bed, to sedate and soothe Her with a good night's sleep before She did any harm to me or anyone else. I told Keith that if he wanted to go out with his friends, that was fine with me.

He replied, "No, I don't really feel like it. I'll stay in with you tonight, love."

An hour later he came into the bedroom, kissed me tenderly, and let me know he changed his mind; he was going out after all. He punctuated that with, "Can I get you anything before I go, sweetie?"

I felt my blood boil. She — my Dark Feminine — was *furious*.

"What?! You're going out? I didn't think you actually would! I just offered that to be nice! If I had known you were going to go out, I would have just stayed at my own house!" I ripped off the covers and leaped out of his bed. Eyes ablaze, I dressed hastily. "I'm going home!" I yelled.

"What?" He retorted, looking genuinely confused. "Why?"

"Never mind," I said under my breath, as my wise Inner SHE attempted damage control.

Too late. The dark, wild woman within had taken over. I stuffed my belongings into my purse and stormed out the door. Keith followed me, trying to figure out what had gone wrong. As many men do, he was focusing on what I had *said* instead of what I was feeling.

"I don't understand," he kept saying. "You told me to go out if I wanted! Now I've gone ahead and made plans. Why are you so upset?"

He was right, of course, but my Dark Feminine had no interest in male rationality. She was raging. But, most of all, that rage was fiercely protecting a hurt and wounded little girl deep inside who was terrified of being abandoned. She no longer felt safe, loved, and wanted.

I was crying. He and I were screaming in the street. I could feel his fear of my emotional intensity.

This man is a Kung Fu master and can kick through walls, I thought. *Why is he afraid of...me?*

His body language grew defensive, his tone hardened, and his heart closed off.

This just made my Inner Little Girl that much more hysterical. It made Her that much more intense.

It didn't end well that night. I went home, as upset as I'd been in months. He went out, angry, confused, and distrustful of me.

Only after much introspection was I eventually able to discern what had occurred that night. During the months and years that have followed, my relationship with Keith has grown tremendously as a result of these kinds of disagreements. Rather than battling my Dark Feminine alone, I have learned to communicate my needs well and to bring Keith on as an ally.

These days, this sort of conflict between us is inconceivable because I know how to express what's really going on under the surface, and Keith has learned how to support my vulnerability. A large part of my work has been helping women to gain this kind of understanding about their own inner darkness so that their partners and families can help support instead of shame and war with them. (We'll explore more about how to do this in the next chapter.)

Facing Your Shadow

Charging out to buy a pack of smokes, even though you "quit." Sitting down with a box of cookies, unable to stop yourself from eating the whole thing. Spacing out on Facebook for two hours, even though you're exhausted. Picking a fight, when what you really want is closeness. These are some of the many ways that our Dark Goddesses, also known as our "shadows," can show up. Our "shadows" represent the part of us that's usually hidden, secretive, and hard to understand. No matter how much we "work" on ourselves, they're still there. Yoga, meditation, positive affirmations, detoxing — none of these seem to help. *"What's wrong with me?!"* we think. Nothing! *Nada*. Our shadows are a normal, useful, and necessary part of being human.

No one is exempt from a shadow, and we never get rid of our shadows. As Ursula K. Le Guin wrote, "When you light a candle, you also cast a shadow."[9] We *all* have little rooms and pockets of shadow in our inner homes. And the more light we shine in the world, the bigger our shadows will be. A truly effective spiritual practice helps us to find these and integrate them with the light of our loving awareness, slowly and patiently, over the course of our entire lives.

"The shadow," a term conceived by Carl Jung, refers to the hidden, unconscious aspects of our psyches. It's our blind spots — those parts of ourselves that we fail to see or know. John Welwood describes our shadow as all of our undigested life experiences.[10] We are all born whole, yet very early on, those parts of ourselves that we are told are "bad" or "unacceptable" slowly get squashed into the cellars of our psyches. Likewise, our brilliant and wonderful aspects also aren't permitted and recognized, so we lock those away too. (We'll explore this "light side" of our shadows in chapter 9.)

As we grow up, our families and cultures insist that we only live out certain parts of our nature. The more polished our personalities (or our egos) become, the more shadow builds up, holding energy equal to our egos. For example, as women, it's okay for us to be polite, but not bitchy. We need to be pretty, but not sexy. It's better to be helpful than selfish. These darker aspects of ourselves never leave or get integrated; they simply get suppressed and compressed in the cellars of our psyches. They become part of our "shadows," the deeply despised parts of ourselves that we don't want anyone to see. Yet as I noted earlier, without recognizing our shadows, we can never be truly alive or empowered, because we are only living out one half of our existence.

Because our psyches want to find equilibrium and our bodies want to move toward health, our shadows will not settle for being locked away forever. In fact, if they stay hidden for long enough, they'll start to take on a life of their own. Then we'll start to act out in ways that feel beyond our control. We'll yell at someone in traffic, cheat on our spouses, binge-eat when everyone in the house has gone to bed, or betray our best friends' trust.

You can identify your shadow behavior because:

1. you're ashamed of it and feel guilty afterward.
2. you feel like you're being "taken over" when you enact it.
3. you often do it in secrecy.

Again, it's important to understand that, when left unattended, our shadows can accumulate even more energy than our egos. When this happens, they threaten to destroy us — and everything that we care about in our lives. We see this in the case of addictions and extreme violence toward ourselves or others. Marion Woodman describes this unconscious shadow material as being like a volcano, gathering a tremendous amount of heat, energy, and intensity under the surface, threatening to erupt all over our cherished light-filled creations at any moment.[11]

Let's learn to utilize the untapped volcanic vitality that's stuck inside our shadows to energize us. How do we release the precious life force trapped inside them? Through conscious, daily shadow work. Without it, we'll perpetually live inside haunted houses, because whatever we can't be with won't let us be. A friend once wisely pointed out that "The Bogey

Man is only the Bogey Man until we turn and face him." Let's take a closer look at our shadows.

Reveal Your Secrets

As the Alcoholics Anonymous adage so astutely states, "We're only as sick as our secrets." Make a list of all of your secrets (don't worry; no one will see this!). What do you do (or what have you *ever* done) that you haven't wanted anyone to see or know about? It can be something as minute as picking your nose in your car or something larger, like stealing something from a department store. Without censorship, write down everything you can remember.

To get the ball rolling, here are some "skeletons in the closet" shared by women in the SHE School:

- Fantasizing about your ex (even though you're married or in a committed relationship)
- Drinking alone to "take the edge off"
- Smoking (even though you're a yoga teacher)
- "Forgetting" to eat
- Falling asleep in bed to Netflix or reruns of TV shows
- Shopping for expensive shoes and clothes
- Indulging in overpriced spa treatments
- Snacking on too many unhealthy sweets and carbs (ice cream, bread and butter)
- Cyber-stalking people on Facebook, Instagram, etc.
- Overscheduling yourself so you set yourself up to fail
- Isolating and retreating into your mind so you don't show up for yourself or anyone around you

Now, without self-condemnation, look over your own list. Everything you've written down is part of your shadow.

Ritualize Your Shadow Behavior

The Dark Goddess *will* emerge as you move toward the light. The bigger your goal, the bigger the obstacles you'll face. Remember that your growing edge always lives within that part of yourself that you can't face.

Your addictions and shadow behavior will always want to resurface when you're in the midst of intense transitions — even if you think you're already healed. You need to be very aware of this truth and work with it skillfully.

The more you create, the more the Dark Goddess will want — and need — to simultaneously destroy. To avoid being annihilated by the Dark Goddess, you must work with her regularly in ritualistic, unthreatening ways, because your unconscious mind doesn't know the difference between real life and ritual. Better to let the Dark Goddess rip in your private, sacred space than all over your beloveds!

Here are a few ways to work with the Dark Goddess:

- Place images of both dark and light feminine archetypes on the altar in your sacred space. Each day feel how they both reside within you. If you don't have a relationship with the archetype of the Dark Feminine, she will continue to appear externally in her deranged form.
- Give expression to the "dark" qualities you listed earlier, in non-damaging ways. *Be* the Dark Feminine through ritual painting, sculpting, drawing, and thrashing around. Tear up and burn your creations.
- Scream in your car, into a pillow, or in the woods. Buy a plastic baseball bat and beat your couch and bed pillows. Stomp your feet into the floor or the earth.
- Make a playlist for your Dark Goddess. Include songs that invoke rage, grief, bitchiness, sluttiness, and self-absorption. Dance to it, feeling the energy of each aspect of her fully.
- Construct a collage of your Dark Goddess. Collect images from magazines that look like her. Place this in your sacred space to help you see her. Or, create a Pinterest board for her. (You can see examples of mine here: www.Pinterest.com/SaraAvantStover.)

Advanced practice: When I was working with my therapist after my bulimia relapse, she suggested that I ritualize my vomiting, which is a wise bodily response to relieve built-up tension throughout the entire core of the body. So, during my morning practice, I would walk mindfully over to the toilet, kneel down, open my mouth, and stick my finger down my throat until I gagged. I never threw up, but I felt relieved nonetheless. This exercise helped me to bring my shadow behavior into the light of day (and my consciousness) by including it in my sacred space. When I didn't make it all bad, it lost its power over me. And while I know my bulimia is a part of me that I'll be in relationship to for the rest of my life, I haven't felt compelled to binge and purge since.

Our judgments about so-called unhealthy foods and habits are often more harmful than the culprits themselves! If your Dark Goddess needs to act out, let her do so with your full consent. The less you judge and shame your behavior, the less harmful it will be in the end. In my own life, I know that the self-hatred I felt after my binge-purge sessions was so much more harmful than the actual act.

Now for some concrete examples of how you can ritualize your shadow behavior. Before you begin, identify the behavior you want to work with. (Note: If you are suffering from the disease of a deep addiction, 100 percent abstinence, with the support of a therapist and/or twelve-step program, is the best path for you.) What takes hold of you so you no longer feel like you have a choice? Whatever that is indicates the doorway. Relinquish self-judgment as you enact these rituals. Do them with your full acceptance whenever you feel drawn to your shadow behavior.

- If you're prone to binge eating, allow yourself to overeat, beyond the point of fullness, during a communal mealtime when you're not emotionally triggered.
- Enjoy a cigarette, allowing each puff to be a prayer you release to the divine.
- Pour yourself your favorite drink. Sit on the front porch and sip it slowly.
- Go out to a club and flirt, gifting someone with your feminine radiance.
- Pop the sleeping pill and feel your body relax and recede into unconsciousness.

I understand that some of these suggestions aren't very nourishing, but your shadow doesn't want you to quit smoking, go on a diet, or drink chamomile tea. She wants to destroy you. So when she arises, rather than judging and shaming yourself, embrace the behavior with at least *partial* acceptance. Ultimately it's your self-compassion — not the Band-Aid of external, healthy habits — that will heal your darkest depths. If the latter worked, we'd all be healed by now.

When we reach for our shadow substances, we're really reaching for the divine. Addictive behavior then becomes thwarted rituals of connection. Native Americans associate tobacco with gratitude and communication between realms. Hindus use sweets, milk, and butter in goddess offerings. Catholics offer wine at mass, and "spirits" have long been seen as a thwarted doorway to "Spirit." All of our shadow acts are desperate, misguided attempts connect with our true Selves, and bringing our shadows into the light of consciousness is our only true path home.

The Danger of Projection

"The enemy is our guru, our teacher," the Dalai Lama teaches.[12] Most of us fear the mess of life, so we blame it on others. As women, we are especially guilty of this. We're so critical of other women! If you doubt this, just read *US Weekly* or watch *E! News* to see the woman bashing that goes on — by other women, no less — after an actress walks the "red carpet gauntlet" at the Academy Awards.

When we don't do daily shadow work, we either judge or idealize those who carry our disowned traits. This is called *projection*. Whenever we feel a strong attraction or repulsion to someone, we know that our shadows are activated and projection is in progress. We will feel triggered by and/or magnetized to these people, over and over and over again until we do the hard work of integrating and assimilating our disowned qualities. Only then can we liberate all the life force we spent on them for ourselves, as Emily Dickinson did when she turned her old love for a man into her new love for life.

With this in mind, one of the ways that we can start to make our shadows conscious, transforming our demons into our daemons, is to look at what we are projecting onto other people. Every relationship serves as a sacred mirror for parts of ourselves we disowned as little girls. Relationships are, therefore, the best — and *only* — way to get to know our shadow. It's usually those closest to us — our spouses, teachers, friends, children, and parents — that we project most of our darkness onto. It's much easier to shame and blame our spouses for being inconsiderate than to acknowledge all the ways that we are too.

To begin, identify your enemies. What do you judge them for? Make a list of all the things you've judged in others over the past week. There's a saying in Tibetan Buddhism that instructs us to "Drive all blames into one." Look at the list and breathe in the recognition that these qualities you're judging in others are actually parts of yourself you haven't been willing to accept. Make a pact to yourself to spend some time in safe, private places to express these qualities and to embrace them as part of who you are.

From this perspective, the people who bother you the most are your most valuable teachers. Take your power back. Own and live out the parts of yourself that you're constantly projecting onto others.

Remember, always take 100 percent responsibility for your experience. When you do this, you can't blame, criticize, or pass the buck onto someone else. You acknowledge that anger, cruelty, and narcissism are all disowned aspects of *yourself*.

A Visualization to Meet
Your Dark Goddess

To listen to this visualization, go to www.TheBookofSHE.com/practices to download the audio file. I've also included it in written form here. Make sure you have your journal and a pen or pencil nearby before you begin.

Come into a comfortable seat. Close your eyes. Take five slow, deep, and even breaths, inhaling for a count of five and exhaling for a count of five. Let your mind follow each breath. Inhale into any physical tension you feel. Exhale, release it. Inhale into any preoccupying emotions. Exhale, release them. Inhale into any thoughts or dominant mind forms. Exhale, release them. Inhale into any sounds or distractions in the room. Exhale, release them. Inhale into your whole body; exhale, release.

Next, get in touch with your earthing cord (from chapter 2). Feel a thick cord extending from your belly down into the center of the earth. Clearly envision each end of the cord. Inhale earth energy up through your feet and legs, as well as through this cord. Exhale and store it in your belly. Breathe in that way a few more times. Then widen and strengthen your earthing cord until you feel a steady flow of surplus earth energy flowing through your body. If at any time you start to feel distracted or overwhelmed during this visualization, reestablish your earthing cord.

Now imagine your inner home. See yourself on the top floor, standing on the staircase landing. Envision the staircase. What kind of a staircase is it? See how this staircase descends all the way down into the cellar of your home.

Place your hand on the railing and slowly walk down, one story, one step at a time. See your surroundings as you go down. What rooms do you pass? How does the light change? How do you feel as you go down through each floor? Now see yourself arriving at the very bottom of the staircase. Is there a cellar door you need to pass through as you do that? Does the temperature and smell of the air shift? Notice what changes as you arrive in the cellar.

See yourself stepping off the very last stair. When you arrive in your cellar, you enter a very dark, dank, disgusting place. Imagine the worst possible cellar that you can — a place you abhor with every fiber of your being. What lives in the cellar that makes you so afraid of going down there? Call forth a place in your mind's eye that represents hell — a place you'd never, ever want to go to.

Do you see it clearly? Bring in all of your senses here. What does it smell like? What's the temperature? Do you hear anything? You can always pause here if you need more time to envision it.

When you've created this space, continue to take slow deep breaths. Now, look to the darkest corner of the cellar. Down on the floor, you see the worst version of yourself possible — who you would be if everything had gone wrong in your life. The more revolting, the better. Allow an image of yourself at your very worst to appear in your mind. Try to sense and see everything about this repulsive version of yourself. How do you look? How do you smell? How do you feel? What are you wearing? What's the look on your face, and in your eyes? What about your hair?

Look more closely. What's something about your lowest self that you didn't see before? Now, step a little closer and say hello. Ask her if she has anything she needs to tell you. Pause and listen. She might speak in words, sounds, movement, symbols, or just a feeling you get from being with her. Again, if you need more time, pause until you feel complete with this step.

Receive what she has to say, and also take some time to ask her any other questions you have for her. When you feel complete, thank her and walk back up the staircase. When you get back to the top, open your eyes, feel the room around you, and fully return from your journey.

Write down what you received from your shadow during your visualization. Write for at least ten minutes without stopping. Keep your pen moving with the stream of your consciousness, describing everything you can remember about your time down in your cellar.

If we can't be with our own pain, there's no way we can be with the pain of others. The more we work with our shadows, the gentler they become and the more we realize just how much we need them to help get us to where we're really wanting to go.

The sooner we embrace the dusty corners of the cellar, the sooner we can truly enjoy the light-filled rooms. We can't actualize our feminine genius without partnering with the Dark Goddess.

Journaling Questions

- What self-sabotaging behaviors keep coming back to haunt you (the ones you've been "working on" for years but can't seem to "get rid of")?
- What are you not able to accept about yourself?
- What is the negative feedback loop that life is currently offering you? What's the wake that your actions are leaving behind you? These both point to your shadow.
- Where are you doing something that doesn't feel like you?
- What do you fear is the worst that could happen if you allow the world to see who you "really" are? Aerate your fears about this.

Chapter 6

Ending the War Within

The challenge for the heroine is not one of conquest
but one of accepting her nameless, unloved parts that have become
tyrannical because she has left them unchecked.

— Maureen Murdock, *The Heroine's Journey*

In the seventh grade, one of my dreams came true: I got to dance in *The Nutcracker* with the New York City Ballet. The perks were endless: dressing with the prima ballerinas backstage, toting home armfuls of flowers every evening, and watching the entire performance — over and over and over again — from the wings. One of my favorite scenes always arrived at the beginning of Act II, in the magical land of the Sugarplum Fairy. A male dancer hiding inside a bonnet floated high up on stilts, which were covered by a humongous, bright yellow, wire-rimmed petticoat skirt. He scuttled out on stage, demurely fanning himself and swaying his "hips." About a quarter through the song, he pulled a string, parted his skirt, and a dozen dancing children ran out from beneath it!

I always remember this image when I think about our inner selves. Although we certainly appear as one person on the outside, when we look inside, we see that we're most definitely *not* a single self. We're a multiplicity — or family — of inner selves, encompassing all of our experiences — past, present, and future. They include our ancestry, gender, nationality, and demon and daemon, representing both our conditioned self and our transcendent Self. They're universal and yet also exist within our individual psyches, influencing our personalities and actions. Some examples of these conditioned inner selves include the Inner Critic, Inner Patriarch, Perfectionist, Protector, Victim, and Vulnerable Child. (We'll explore the transcendent inner selves in chapter 9.) Teasing each inner self apart, getting to know both the capacities and the limitations of each, we see that our shadows aren't some amorphous, dark blobs in our psyches. Our shadows actually represent a continually evolving *process* comprised of a conglomeration of a lot of different qualities and subpersonalities.

Humanizing the inner voices that comprise our shadows releases them from their false dominion over our lives. When we're masters over, rather than victims to, our demons, we understand that we possess far more greatness than we ever imagined. Our wise, transcendent inner selves often get buried underneath our incessant, usually violent, inner chatter. Yet the more we get to know our inner selves, cultivating relationships of open communication, honesty, safety, and trust with them, the more easily we'll be able to mobilize all of our inner resources in service of birthing the lives we most desire. Therefore, to become whole women, we need to create strong and flexible egos by cultivating harmony among all of our inner selves. Only through restoring order in our inner homes can we experience genuine inner peace. Getting what we want out of life is a tall order; to succeed, we're going to need to rally *every* aspect of our inner selves to get on board this noble cause.

As I was growing up, my mother often said, "Sara, you are your own worst enemy." She was right! When left unchecked, some of my inner selves used to speak to me far more savagely than I would ever dare speak to *anyone*. I now see that this is true for *every* woman I work with. It's much easier to see the wars in current affairs than the ones being waged within us, but we are *all*, without a doubt, our own worst enemies.

When left unchecked, our more diabolical inner selves team up to become the dreaded demons we explored in the previous chapter, making us feel forever damaged, wrong, and unworthy of love. When we don't know how to be the masters of our own minds, our minds act like naughty children and our shadows take over. They do whatever they want, wreaking havoc by allowing our disowned selves to run the show. Fatigue, low libido, autoimmune disorders, and depression can all be symptoms of our disowned selves battling one another and draining our energy.

It's important to note that this epidemic is only growing worse as the time we spend on technology increases. Studies show that our moods plummet toward anxiety and depression the more we spend time online.[1] When we're busy tweeting and checking our Facebook feeds, we're constantly comparing ourselves to others rather than listening to and trusting our own inner wisdom. When we zone out to surf the Web, we're not resting in our spacious awareness, and our bully inner selves sneak in and take over. Unless we train our minds to rest in the present moment, through daily periods of kindhearted mindfulness meditation *and* active communication with our inner selves, we will become more and more disconnected from our *highest* Selves.

This latter piece, dialoguing with our inner voices, truly holds the key to stopping the civil war within. In order to reclaim the throne of our inner temples as fully functioning, free women, we need to become loving mothers to *all* of our inner selves. *In fact, the work in this chapter always proves to be the most pivotal piece of this journey for women.*

Contrary to popular practice and belief, we do not approach these inner voices with aggression. We're not trying to fix, beat up, or "get rid" of these inner voices. It's simply not effective to tell them to "shut up" or "get the hell away," or to lock them in a closet until the end of time. You can never heal what you criticize. What you resist persists! Instead, we must learn to treat ourselves with love and compassion.

To begin the practice of cultivating loving kindness for our inner enemies, we can call upon the qualities of motherhood we explored in chapter 3 and attune to *all* of our inner selves, giving each contact and space. A mother doesn't simply listen to one child and always ignore the other. That would be a disaster! Instead, to be mothers who create a nourishing home for *all* of our children, let's take time to get to know each one equally. What do they look like? Sound like? What are their names? Their needs? Their deepest motives? At the end of the day, we *all* want to feel seen, heard, loved, and valued. We want to know that we belong and that it's okay for us to exist. Our inner selves are no exception to this.

Guess who deserves the spotlight first? The dynamic duo that most consistently sabotages our happiness, health, and success — the Inner Critic and the Vulnerable Child.

The Inner Critic

"Don't you dare take up all that space!"

"Nobody cares what you think."

"You don't know enough yet."

"Fatty! You can't wear that!"

"You're such a horrible person — rotten to the core."

"If you do that, everyone will know how stupid you really are."

Ouch. Sound familiar? These are some of the *many* ways that we may experience our Inner Critics, or ICs. The ICs live within each of us — men and women, young and old. Their virulence spreads around the entire world, sparing no one, no matter how "evolved," "spiritual," or "mature" anyone claims to be. When we don't do our inner work, our Inner Critics get *way* out of hand. Yet when we do, they can, quite surprisingly, become great allies on our paths. Since awareness always opens the door to healing, let's explore how our ICs first developed.

When our parents, caretakers, or teachers scolded, judged, or shamed us, our psyches quickly realized that we needed *some* form of protection to survive, so our ICs stepped in. They first arose by internalizing the very messages that our authority figures voiced to try to keep us in line. The more judgment we were exposed to as children, the stronger our own ICs will be (and the stronger our Inner Judges will be — that part of ourselves that criticizes others, for this is the outer function of our Inner Critics).

The Inner Critics quickly realized that in order to survive in our homes, and to spare us shame and pain, they needed to constantly remind us of those things that our parents told us. Anything that might be inappropriate or threatening to our families was immediately suppressed, and eventually disowned, for expressing it could have risked our very survival. To keep us in line and to stop us from rocking the boats of our familial status quos, our Inner Critics are always asking, "What will other people think?" Our ICs want us to fit in. They want the world to like us, and they are willing to do whatever they can to make sure that happens. *No matter how hard we try, we can never please our Inner Critics.*

As we grow older, our ICs can take over our psyches like parasites when left unchecked. They block our creativity, prevent us from experiencing pleasure, and keep us from sharing our gifts with the world. As a result, we become depressed, haunted with the malaise that we're never good enough, there's something wrong with us, and we're too ordinary and need to be more "unique" and "special."

The unceasing discontent of our ICs often leads us to acts of self-sabotage. When besieged by Inner Critic attacks, we may compulsively feel the need to tune out by procrastinating, smoking, overworking, drinking, taking drugs, shopping, watching TV, surfing the Internet, masturbating, binging, purging, or overexercising. Such avalanches of negative feelings signal us that we've left our Inner Critics unchecked. They've sneaked into the role of despots of our inner households. When we realize this, then we can take steps to bring the true masters — our *SHEs* — back into place.

What brings on these IC attacks? External criticism, lack of sleep, and stress. They can also come on when we drink too much, eat foods that don't agree with us, enter an uncomfortable or unfamiliar setting, or struggle through certain times of the day or night when we feel more vulnerable or are on the brink of a breakthrough. For women, Inner Critic attacks can also come when we're experiencing PMS, during certain other phases of the hormonal cycle (especially during perimenopause, pregnancy, and early motherhood), and during the darker times of the year. These causes help us see another reason why deep self-understanding is so essential.

As bleak as all this sounds, there's still hope for us. Instead of behaving like a petulant child under the auspices of an oppressive parent, let's take the reins back and become the *conscious* parent in every situation. Recognize that the Inner Critics' hostility is coming out of fear that you are going to fail. This is the best way they know how to protect you, and they often just need to be reassured that you're in charge and on top of the situation.

Eleven Steps to Transforming Your Inner Critic

Like all of your inner selves, your IC is a constantly evolving aspect of your ego. For this reason, you need to work with it (daily!) for the rest of your life. Think of this act as psychic dental flossing. Without doing this inner work, your inner home rots and decays. I know it can seem like a lot at first, but as you start to get more used to it, it becomes second nature — like talking to your dog, child, or spouse.

1. Understand that your IC is NOT you.

Your Inner Critic is a part of your small, conditioned self and a result of childhood programming. It developed at a young age in order to ensure your survival by adopting the messages of your caregivers.

2. Identify the signs that your IC has taken over and you're having an Inner Critic attack.

In her book *Playing Big*, women's leadership expert Tara Sophia Mohr highlights eleven universal qualities of our ICs' voices.[2] Watch out for mental scripts such as the following (all of which are quoted from *Playing Big*):

- "Harsh, rude, mean"
- "Binary" (black-and-white thinking)
- "Ostensibly, the voice of reason" (seems to always be arguing for your own best interest)
- "The voice of 'You aren't ready yet'"
- "The voice of 'You aren't good at math/negotiation/technical stuff'"
- "The voice of body perfectionism"
- "The tape" (repeating thoughts, a.k.a. your "IC's Greatest Hits")
- "A broken record" (has been saying the same thing for decades)
- "Irrational but persistent"
- "The one-two punch" ("attacks you with critical thoughts, and then shames you for having those thoughts")
- "The inner critic may take inspiration from critical people in your life" (hearing "echoes of a parent, sibling, or boss in your inner critic's voice")

As well, it's important to note the *emotional* cues. What do you feel when you're having an IC attack? Anxious? Overwhelmed? Make a list of the dominant emotions to get clear of the effects.

Along the same lines, learn to recognize the *physical* cues. What are the corresponding bodily sensations and ensuing shadow behavior when you're under attack? Do you feel tightness somewhere? The urge to harm yourself or another in some way? Knowing these symptoms will help you recognize when you're under attack.

3. Name that you're having an Inner Critic attack.

Admit this to yourself. Tell a friend or spouse via text, email, or phone call. For instance, when a member of our SHE School community was having an IC attack, she shared the following message in our online forum.

> "My inner critic can be so fatalistic! You'll *never* do this....
> You'll *never* be this.... You'll *never* achieve this...."

Simply voicing this in the presence of others freed her from being tormented by her IC. *Acknowledging and naming something diminishes its power over you.*

4. Externalize its messages.

Write down exactly what you hear your Inner Critic saying to you. List it all on a piece of paper. Then rip it up or burn it to externalize and release the violence you would otherwise feel inclined to express internally. Alternately, role-play with a friend. Have your friend represent you while you personify your Inner Critic.

5. Pause and listen to your "IC's Greatest Hits."

Write down what your IC says to you over and over and over again. This will help you recognize the thought patterns behind your IC attacks.

6. Understand how the Inner Critic came to be and generate compassion for it.

Do the messages of your IC sound familiar? Where have you heard these before? Here are some insights that women in our SHE School had about the roots of their ICs' messages.

> "I realized that my Inner Critic has my father's voice! That's exactly how he used to talk to me."

> "My IC [tells me] not be as big, to quiet my energy down, to be smaller and less radiant. My mom gave me these messages. Her body is fairly closed down, and she is very afraid of her own aliveness."

7. Personify your IC.

Is it male or female? What does it look like? How old is it? What does it sound like? Give it a name. Draw a picture of it. Here's another example from our group.

> "I imagine my Inner Critic has her hair tightly pulled back in a bun with a pen holding it up. She looks put-together and proper, with a pencil skirt and tucked-in blouse."

8. Share with those you trust what your Inner Critic sounds and looks like.

Through this process, we let go of the belief that we're terminally unique. We're not the only ones embroiled in this inner civil war! Through sharing, we learn that all of our Inner Critics sound *exactly* alike.

9. Make a daily date with your IC.

These dates are especially important when you're in transition; are feeling sensitive, vulnerable, or depleted; or are prone to more external evaluation than usual. When your IC is concerned, daily contact with it isn't a luxury, it's a necessity. Even if you think you've already "healed" your IC, you need to keep up with this too. Remember, your IC is a master shape shifter. Its job is to criticize, and it will always find new and better ways to excel and criticize you!

To begin this work, speak to the IC's voice in your head. Write the dialogue in your journal. Allow your IC to speak to you by writing with your nondominant hand. Include it in your four-part check-in (from chapter 3) to see what it's saying and what it needs. Tell it what your plans are for the day. Ask for its opinion. Consider its response. Then allow your word to be the final word. From there, give your IC any clear direction, clarification, or pacification, as needed. Be a firm, yet loving, mother to your Inner Critic!

10. Meditate daily to keep your mind strong and healthy.

Strengthen your undistracted attention, within an atmosphere of loving kindness, to become the observer of your thoughts and emotions. The more you see that these are fluid, ever-changing energies, the more you can remain the master of your mind and inner domain through knowing the truth: They aren't "you."

11. Understand your IC's job, don't slack on *your* job, and dialogue with its related inner selves.

Your IC's job is to protect your vulnerability. Period. That's its deepest motive behind everything it does. If your IC is being especially loud, it means it's working overtime to protect your Vulnerable Child. Ultimately, this is your job, not the job of your IC. An IC attack is your signal to step up and mother your Inner Child.

Our Inner Critics took the lead when we were little girls in order to protect our vulnerability. They jumped in because *someone* had to keep guard! Now that you're a grown woman, you can step in for the IC and send it off for a much-needed vacation. Do this by working with your Vulnerable Child directly. Trust me, your Inner Critic is just as tired of doing this job as you are of having the IC step up to the plate again and again!

Reclaiming your role as the adult in charge is a win-win-win scenario. When you become a good mother to your Vulnerable Child, your Inner

Critic starts to soften and relax. Simultaneously, you come closer to living from the true feminine strength it's been faithfully guarding all along.

The Vulnerable Child

Adorning the staircases and doorways of Buddhist temples across Thailand, fierce demons, in the form of water dragons called *nagas*, stand guard. I always bow internally to these monsters as I pass by them to such sacred spaces, because I know that their motive is not to harm me, but to protect the immeasurable treasures the temple contains. The same holds true within us. Every fierce demon safeguards an even more precious *daemon* — including the daemon of tender, trembling vulnerability.

In her book *Daring Greatly*, Brené Brown writes, "Vulnerability is the birthplace of love, belonging, joy, courage, empathy, and creativity. It is the source of hope, empathy, accountability, and authenticity. If we want greater clarity in our purpose or deeper and more meaningful spiritual lives, vulnerability is the path."[3] Sadly, we live in a world that dismisses vulnerability, the most feminine of all human qualities. As a result, your number one disowned self is probably your Vulnerable Child. For women, this is a *major* hitch in the pursuit of feminine power. We've learned to armor and shield those aspects of ourselves that society labels as weak, high maintenance, embarrassing, or overdramatic. Instead of celebrating our softness we "put on our big girl pants" in order to "be strong."

If we're excluding our own vulnerability, no amount of confidence-boosting techniques or fancy conferences can help us find our power. We have to heal the source — not just intellectually, but *experientially*, *every single day*. Here's a quick look at a catalyst that prompted me to more deeply examine this piece of myself.

A while back, Keith and I hosted a party in our new home. Despite my mother's long-standing warning that "expectation is premeditated disappointment," a part of me held a deep longing that Keith would toast me — declaring his love and appreciation in front of our closest friends and family. I offered something similar to Keith at a party I threw for him on his fortieth birthday a couple of years ago, and somehow I just assumed he would think to reciprocate. Therefore, I never shared this need and longing with him. *Bad idea.* Despite my best attempts to coach myself to release my expectations on the days leading up to the party, a sneaky, small part of myself just couldn't let it go.

I think we all know how this story ends. Keith *didn't* toast me, and I went to sleep that night feeling unloved, unseen, and unappreciated — even though it was a beautiful evening and he shared his love for me in his own way.

A few days later, I was still upset. On a phone call with one of my mentors, I recounted what had happened. I shared that I knew something deeper was at play because, no matter how hard I tried to rationalize my way out of my self-pity and disappointment, I just couldn't snap out of it. My mentor then shone a light into a place I least expected — my Vulnerable Child. (I call her "Sarie Bear," for that's what my grandmother affectionately called me when I was little.)

Almost immediately after we turned our attention toward Sarie Bear, an old memory surfaced. In the summer when I was about six, not long after my youngest sister was born, I was feeling lonely and neglected. My father was traveling a lot, and my mother was overwhelmed with taking care of me and my three sisters, all under the age of eight. One afternoon I headed out to a poison ivy patch in the woods beside our house. Knowing I was *highly* allergic, I picked up a shiny red-and-green marbled leaf and rubbed it all over my face and arms. I woke up the next day with my eyes swollen shut and my fingers puffed up like walrus flippers. Despite my discomfort, I secretly relished that I could spend the week in my mom's bed, the center of her attention for a cherished short while.

With my mentor I saw something shocking: My *entire* life was built upon moments like these. Most of them weren't as extreme as rubbing poison ivy all over my body, but the pattern of pushing and hurting myself in exchange for love and attention — from working too hard, to asserting my agenda in the world in a way that was inauthentic, to exercising when I was tired — ran through my entire life in different degrees. *Every single instance rooted back to that little girl who just wanted to be loved.* At our party, Sarie Bear was the one who was hurt because Keith didn't acknowledge her — not me. She thought his praise would make her feel better, even though, deep down, it never, ever would. My mentor reminded me that *I'm* the only one who can ever fill the gaping hole Sarie Bear feels in her heart. I'm the only one who can *ever* give her the love she needs. It's my job to love her, see her, praise her, meet her needs, and slowly help her grow up.

"You'll be surprised," my mentor joked. "The more you give your little girl what she needs, the more Keith — and the world — will inadvertently start giving you the praise you've been seeking. You don't do the practice with that as the motivation, but the truth is, that's how it will turn out."

Although I had been working with Sarie Bear for years already, it was time to go deeper. I commenced what I now lovingly refer to as "The Sarie Bear Sadhana."

The Sarie Bear Sadhana

(*Sadhana* means "spiritual practice" in Sanskrit.)

Find a picture of yourself before the age of eight. Place it on the nightstand beside your bed. Recall a nickname from that time in your life. That's what you'll now call your Inner Little Girl, which is how I'll now refer to your Vulnerable Child.

Before you get out of bed each morning for the next ninety days, look at the picture of your little-girl self, until it becomes so vivid that you can see her in your imagination with your eyes closed. Turn to her in your mind's eye and see what she's doing. What position is she in? Is she engaged in an activity? Can you tell, just from watching, how she's doing today?

Say good morning and greet her. Tousle her hair, hug her, or do whatever feels appropriate. Look at her with your full attention. Tell her, "I'm here. I see you." Then ask her, "How are you?" and "What do you need?"

Listen to her responses. Don't get out of bed until you register a clear answer from her. Commit to giving her what she needs that day, without fail.

Note: This practice only takes a few minutes, and it *will* change your life. When you first begin, don't be alarmed if your Inner Little Girl doesn't want to talk. When I started working with Sarie Bear a decade ago, she was crouched in a ball in the corner of my childhood closet, sobbing. With your daily, loving presence, this will start to shift for you. Give it time.

More Ways to Work with Your Inner Little Girl

- Dialogue with her through writing. For years, this was how I communicated with Sarie Bear. Ask her questions with your dominant hand, and then let her answer them with your weak hand. Since this child usually recedes within us before the age of eight, she holds your essence and your capacity to be deeply intimate with all of life. Within her lives your creativity, passion, sense of wonder, awe, and magic. She also carries your most evolved intuitive capacities in her ability to be exquisitely aware of everything around her. She holds within her the treasures that you are seeking. Her answers are usually so right-on and surprising!

- Where in your life can you see your Inner Little Girl acting out? What are you currently seeking love, praise, and attention for?

Now when I attune to Sarie Bear, she's often drawing, playing with her toys, or watching cartoons on the couch. Sometimes she's sleeping, cuddled up next to me. Other times, usually when I'm under stress and have been very busy, I see she is visibly distressed. She'll feel anxious and abandoned when Keith leaves the house to run errands or when I go to a noisy party. Usually her needs are incredibly simple: to have a smoothie for breakfast, go to a dance class, take a walk outside, eat pizza for dinner, drink hot chocolate, take a nap, go to the movies.

When I ask her what she needs, and then give it to her, every day, I honor my own sensitivity. Rather than overriding that part of myself, I acknowledge and partner with it. This simple practice has radically shifted how I show up in all areas of my life — my intimate relationship, work, self-care, and social interactions. Now I don't go a day without doing it, because, if I do, my attention gets misguided and I start looking for validation externally.

I recommend working with just the Inner Critic and Inner Little Girl every day, through the methods offered earlier in this chapter, for ninety days. Then, as you get very well acquainted with them, move on to explore more members of your inner family, such as the ones discussed next.

The Inner Patriarch

Having gone to one of the most feminist colleges in the world — Columbia University's all-women's Barnard College, in New York City — I've always considered myself to be progressive. *I'm a strong, smart woman. I can do whatever I want to do.* What I didn't realize, however, was that even though I did have opportunities to learn and express myself in ways that my mother didn't, I still allowed the patriarch within to direct my life through unconscious, mental programming that constantly held me back.

Just as our Inner Critics developed to protect us from the shame and pain of disgracing our families, our Inner Patriarchs developed to protect us from dishonoring our societies. To keep us in line, we internalized the voices that told us we were inferior to men:

"You must be seen and not heard!"
"You'll have to work twice as hard as a man in order to earn half as much."
"No matter how hard you try, you'll always be inferior to men."

It can be quite disorienting and humbling when we finally catch on to the damage our Inner Patriarchs are actually doing to us. Oppression hasn't just been happening "out there"; it's been happening under own roofs! Here are some of the qualities of your Inner Patriarch:

- Demands success at all costs
- Thinks your feelings and vulnerability are "weak"
- Scoffs at your intuition
- Requires scientific proof for every instinctive point you make in order for it to be considered real and valid
- Prizes the reason and rationality of the mind above all else
- Dominates, controls, and conquers
- Always puts "me" first
- Denigrates nature and your body

Working with Your Inner Patriarch

1. Write down all the negative beliefs and criticisms that you harbor —
    or that you've been exposed to — about being a woman. Consider
    the messages you've received from:

    *   your mother
    *   your father
    *   your grandparents
    *   your teachers (male and female)
    *   movies, TV, and magazines
    *   pornography
    *   past partners and lovers
    *   religious figures

2. Understand that your Inner Patriarch is a mighty force, since it's a
    conglomeration of some of your other domineering inner selves,
    including your Inner Critic and Perfectionist (along with more sub-
    personalities that we aren't exploring here, like the Pusher, Con-
    troller, and Comparer). The more you can parse out these distinct
    voices, the more you'll be able to work effectively with your Inner
    Patriarch.

The Perfectionist

As little girls, many of us grew up believing that so long as we were perfect, we would be loved. Somewhere along the way, we probably adopted
dangerous beliefs such as "I am what I accomplish" and "As long as I look
pretty, I will be loved."

Perfectionism yanks our invisible corsets too tight and clamps down
our unique creative expression. It stops failure and mess in their tracks,
and in doing so, denies both life and death. Perfectionism is, at its core,
about control. It's trying to earn external approval while diminishing our
inner self-worth. It constantly tells us we're not okay how we are and we
"shouldn't be feeling this way." It keeps us from finishing — or even getting started on — those things that we feel most called to create.

Working with Your Perfectionism

- When you're in a sticky situation, write in your journal to reflect on what you would do if you trusted yourself fully and knew you didn't have to do it perfectly.
- Contemplate whether or not your Perfectionist sounds like anyone you know.
- Follow the lead of one of my teachers, Sarah Powers, and ask yourself what it would look like for you to be perfectly willing to accept your imperfections.
- In any moment when you're giving of yourself and feeling compelled to push, ask inwardly, "Can this be enough right now? Can *I* be enough right now?"

What if *good* really is *good enough*? Acknowledge that you're trying your best. If you can get out of your own way and avoid your usual methods of pushing and forcing, then you can lean on your innate inner gifts to forge the way. Let it be easy!

Note: If you have a strong Perfectionist, then your more relaxed selves may have gone into shadow (e.g., your "boundary setters," "party girls," "beach bums," and "slobs"). In order to find greater harmony and balance in your life, you'll need to revive these disowned selves and learn to turn down the dial on the voice of your Perfectionist.

Some Final Notes on Working with Your Inner Selves

Inner unrest is a sign that you need to pause and pay attention to one (or many) of your precious inner selves — both the dominant *and* the disowned ones. Just as you get more and more upset if someone isn't seeing, hearing, or acknowledging you (or if someone is verbally abusing you), your inner selves experience this too. Here are some final directions to guide your way.

- You can work with all of your inner selves with the same techniques you used in "Eleven Steps to Transforming Your Inner Critic" on pages 125–29.
- Be gentle and patient. If you start to feel overwhelmed while working with these voices, slow down and ease up.
- Don't ever do this work alone! These inner selves function in relationship to one another. Therefore, you usually need external relationships to help you see these jumbled-up parts of your inner landscape with more accuracy. In most cases, it's best to begin this work with another person, such as a mentor or therapist. This empathic other can serve as the mediator between your inner selves until your ego is strong enough to do it for you.
- Remind yourself that there's no finish line here. These cycles of growth continue throughout our entire lives. Even if you get to the place where you can mediate between your inner selves on your own, when new pockets of undigested material and disowned selves emerge inside, you'll need to go back to your mentor or therapist so that someone else can once again help hold space for you.
- Note that these inner selves can be devious! Even if you express your party girl or beach bum, she too might be disowned if you let her leak out in unskillful ways. Does her partying or slacking off support or undermine your deepest intentions? If it's the latter, you've disowned her by letting her act out without your sovereign command.

Remember, if one of your inner selves is making a lot of noise...

- Don't tell it to shut up.
- Don't ignore it.
- Don't push it away.
- Hear it out and see whom it's protecting.
- Give it some time in the spotlight.
- Be a good mother to your inner family. Give everyone a seat at the table of your life.

If you want inner peace, becoming attentive to your inner needs is the path. As you progress, you will free yourself from the limiting patterns that sabotage your life's goals and dreams.

Now, in the depths of the underworld, look around. Do you feel more at ease? More oriented and adjusted to the murky black? From this place, you're ready to fully see how to transmute the darkness of your warring inner selves into wisdom. You're approaching the tipping point — the place of magic and miracles.

Journaling Questions

- How have you related to your inner family up until now? Does this mirror anything from your family of origin or your family life now? What do you notice here?
- What are the top three ways that you'll explore working with your Inner Critic and Inner Little Girl for the next ninety days?
- Can you recall any life experiences when your Inner Patriarch or Perfectionist took over? What was the result of that?
- When you tune into what your Inner Little Girl needs right now, what do you discover? How is she feeling *right now*?

Chapter 7

*Unlocking the Magic
in Your SHE Cycles*

> Woman is a very, very strong being. Magical.
> That's why I am afraid of women.
>
> — Carl Jung,
> C. G. Jung, Emma Jung, and Toni Wolff:
> A Collection of Remembrances

It was quite peculiar, what happened that weekend. Now I know: that's just what feminine magic looks like. Thirty of us sat in the opening circle of my Mother's Day retreat at Kripalu Center for Yoga & Health in Lenox, Massachusetts. During each woman's turn to hold the "talking stick," she shared her name and her intention for coming. Halfway through, Margeritte took the stick. Sitting a few inches outside the circle, she stayed silent for several moments. Her shoulders hunched forward, causing her wavy, red hair to hide most of her pale face. Then she began to speak very quietly, her words validating what her body had already revealed.

"I didn't want to come here this weekend," she murmured. "My daughter gave this to me as a Mother's Day gift. She told me I needed to come."

Margerrite's eyes stayed fixated on a patch of gray carpet in front of her. "My eldest son died in a car accident four months ago today. I've hardly been able to get out of bed since. It took *a lot* for me to come here."

We all took a deep breath with — and for — her.

"That's all I have to share right now," she concluded. Then she appeared to recede back into numb invisibility.

The next morning I led the women through a three-hour yoga and meditation practice. We journaled about our relationships to our mothers and the Mother. We meditated, concentrating our attention in our belly centers and breathing into, visualizing, and dialoguing with our wombs. Throughout, I kept a close eye on Margeritte. She had set up her mat in the back of the room, but to my surprise, despite her limited yoga experience, she fullheartedly participated in every pose I offered.

On the final morning of our retreat, however, Margeritte was nowhere to be found. I led our closing circle and enjoyed lunch with the group before we departed. Still no Margeritte. Then, as I was on my way up to my room to retrieve my luggage, someone called my name from behind. Turning around, I saw a smiling woman who seemed to beam like the day's spring sun. *Who is this person?* I thought to myself.

"Sara! It's Margeritte!" she exclaimed, walking toward me. My jaw unhinged in shock.

"Margeritte?! Are you okay? What happened?" I reached my arms out to hug her.

She explained that after our womb-centered practices, she started to have what felt like labor pains (even though she was postmenopausal). She continued to experience quasi-contractions, so just after midnight her roommate called an ambulance, which brought her to the emergency room. The doctors could find no trace of a problem, but to be safe, they kept her overnight. For the next several hours, Margeritte breathed with the pain in her womb, releasing what seemed to be endless streams of tears. The next morning she not only felt 100 percent fine, but she also felt relieved of the thick, icy grief she'd been frozen under since the day her son died. She felt alive again.

"I just need to thank you, Sara," Margeritte shared, wiping tears away. "I have no idea what exactly happened last night, but it was like my son was the one who wanted me to come here this weekend. He knew it was time for me to let go and get on with my life again. To do that, I guess I needed to fully release the grief from my womb. I feel like I just gave birth — to myself. This has been a Mother's Day in the truest and most unexpected ways."

The Holy Spirit in Your Creative Organs

How does this magic, the Mother's magic, work, exactly? Just as it's impossible to know exactly what causes a baby to grow from an embryo or an oak tree to grow from an acorn, your creative capacity remains a deep mystery that you can never fully grasp with your mind. Yet your body communicates these wisdoms constantly, because as a woman, you carry the Divine Feminine within your anatomy. Way down in the root of your femininity, in your pelvic bowl, reside the jewels of your inner temple — your womb, ovaries, and yoni. These gems allow you to cocreate miracles with the divine. They're the seat of your intuition, your personal portal to the metaphysical, and the throne of your SHE. They enact your capacity to fulfill the infinite creative potential of the Goddess within your very finite body. Within the sacred cycles of creation — receiving and releasing — in your creative organs, you access the exact inner tools you need to transmute your demons into your daemons. You then become the magic wand that can transform obstacles into opportunities.

As we move forward, please know that this chapter is for *every* woman in *any* season of life, whether or not...

- your cycles are regular and "normal."
- you suffer irregular, painful, or missing cycles.
- you want to have a child (or just had one).
- you're perimenopausal, menopausal, or postmenopausal.

Important: *No woman can afford to skip this step!* Your cycles are the *key* that turns your Heroine's descent into her ascent. Without participating in them in the way I'll describe here, you will not experience your Heroine's homecoming. Here's how *every* woman can participate.

- If you've had your womb or ovaries removed, you can still call upon the energy of your creative organs. Just as someone who has had a leg removed still feels its presence as a "phantom limb," your creative organs, once removed, still hold the essence of their subtle energy functions.

- Likewise, whenever I speak about our *physical* menstrual cycles, if you aren't currently menstruating, follow the lunar cycle to participate.

Please hold these perspectives throughout the next two chapters and participate accordingly.

Root, Womb, and Yoni Breathing

Breathe now into the vulnerable space between your pubic bone and belly button. If it's hard for you to feel this part of your body, employ your imagination and visualize it. Where your attention goes, energy flows. Place a hand there as you're reading — either directly on your lower belly or, if you feel comfortable, cupped gently around the base of your body, something we all naturally did as little girls to help us feel safe and rooted to the earth. Breathe into your root (or your pelvic floor), your womb, and your ovaries. Allow your yoni to also breathe, feeling a pulsation of expansion and contraction in the lips of your vagina and the entire base of your body. Notice any feelings or judgments that arise as you read these words. Invite them all to be here. Everything's welcome. Stay with the process. Please continue to invite this region of your body into your experience of reading this chapter — both mentally and, most important, through your feeling awareness.

Our bodies' creative cycles make *all* women master artists and have *everything* to do with *all parts of our lives*. Our cycles, through both our periods and our connection to the moon and the earth's seasons, are how our souls evolve during our lifetimes through continual rhythms of death and rebirth. Because they allow us to be emissaries in direct communication with the Mother Goddess, I call them our "SHE Cycles." These include our hormonal cycles, but also transcend those elements to embrace both our much larger visionary, creative capacities as women *and* our divine nature.

Your Sacred Anatomy

Your sacred anatomy — and all the deep, feminine strength and wisdom it brings through your SHE Cycles — is your womanly birthright. However, most of us carry ancient tension and numbness in our pelvises, and these interfere with allowing our true feminine strength to fully flow through and nourish us. Participating in our SHE Cycles helps to melt this tension, release our true creative fire, and keep us vibrant and growing, at any age.

Your Uterus

Like the ocean and moon, our wombs ebb and flow, wax and wane, in their own patterns, building and shedding their uterine linings each month and working synergistically with our ovaries. The Mother and your connection to the earth live in your womb. *This is the seat of your creative potential as a woman.* Here reside your true voice, the song that you came to this world to sing, and your intuition. Your womb also serves as the storehouse for past grief — both personal, collective, and ancestral. This is the vessel within which you directly comanifest with spirit and heal your lineage. It exhibits a centripetal pull, as feminine/yin power magnifies things *in*.

Your Ovaries

Like little bonfires, your ovaries emit innocent radiance, which has never been and can never be tainted and doesn't need to be contrived or cultivated externally. They also house your soft, receptive, yet fierce feminine strength — the antidote to pushing and overexertion, our usual modes of expressing power. Full of wonder, they face uncertainty with courage, remembering that *anything* is possible.

Whether or not you consider yourself an artist, each of your eggs holds the seed for a new creative project — a baby, a bucket-list excursion, or, in my case, this book! Creativity isn't something that happens "out there" in certain areas of your life; it happens right here in your body.

Your Yoni/Vagina

Serving as the hallway between your womb and the world, your yoni releases old physical, psychic, and emotional debris each month through the shedding of your uterine lining. It also draws in pleasure and fertility, through orgasms and semen, and serves as the threshold into new life during birth. It's the transitory, preparatory portal between the cosmic void and the light of the manifest world. Regain vibrancy here by *consciously choosing* what you let in, what you birth, and what you let go of.

Reversing Our "Curse"

One of the most profound sources of our spiritual insight and feminine power is the very thing that we, as women, are taught to hide or ignore. I like to say it's the m's — our menarche and menopause, menses and moods.

We have learned to take ownership of many of our uniquely feminine gifts, yet the roots of our femininity, our cycles, are still remarkably pushed to the side. When they're spoken of, it's as something that seems separate from us and needs to be managed, or something to be singled out and discussed apart from our larger femininity. Despite all the advances we've made in the field of feminine empowerment over the past century, our cycles, and our bodies in general, remain our final frontier.

In fact, just as many of us learned to ignore our Inner Little Girls, for centuries we have been taught to disown our cycles — and along with them, the daemons they contain and protect. This misguided view of womanhood dates all the way back to the Inquisition in the early 1200s, when patriarchal rule began to dominate and suppress more land-based matriarchal goddess cultures. At that time, a woman's cycles became feared and defiled. Powerful men began to pronounce that menstruating women were evil witches, belonging to the devil, and were to be avoided at all costs. They claimed that approaching women during this time would cause men to lose their vitality, wisdom, and strength. As a result, women began to be shunned during their menses. They were forbidden to look at the sun, speak to a man, or enter sacred spaces. Thus, what began as a maneuver for power grew into truth.

Whereas a woman's menstrual blood was once thought to be so potent that it could fertilize crops if a woman bled on the fields, now men believed that it would destroy fruits, sour wine, rust iron, and cloud mirrors. Even twentieth-century anthropologists encouraged menstrual taboos by describing women as "out of order," "suffering from monthly illness," or "stricken with the malady common to their sex."[1] The Catholic Church still prohibits the ordination of women, and one of the reasons cited is that a menstruating priestess would "pollute" the altar.[2]

Sadly, we all still carry many of these judgments about our own cycles today. They persist in tampon and pad commercials: "Now you can be the same every day of the month." We're urged to hide and deny our cycles. No wonder we see them as a nuisance.

To heal this, let's recognize the division and explore an alternate paradigm for our full, feminine emancipation. We need to reclaim the ancient knowing that our cycles offer us each direct access to the mind and heart of the Goddess. *We can't know the Divine Feminine without being intimate with our cycles.* Our cycles are our hotlines to the holy, and when we participate in them, we all become mystics.

Like many women, I used to think of my SHE Cycles as a nuisance: something to "put up with" each month. Years of being on birth control pills made me feel disconnected from my cycle, my intuition, and my overall sense of being a woman. I denied my body's messages, and suffered physical and emotional consequences (severe cervical dysplasia, ovarian cysts, anxiety, depression, insomnia, eating disorders, irregular menstruation). Finally, after years of study and deep inner work, I reconnected to my cycles — and was astonished to discover within them a wellspring of creativity, intuition, and embodied wisdom. When I got off the Pill and my cycles returned after an absence of several years, I realized that my SHE Cycles held the key to my healing. It turns out that when we live in harmony with our cycles, our world gets a whole lot easier.

You see, your SHE Cycle isn't a "curse." It's an alchemical miracle, hiding in plain sight, happening right in your own body. And if you learn to work with it (not against it), you'll be amazed at the creativity and strength you'll find there. I want to forever change the way you see and live with your cycles, because they have *everything* to do with your power and happiness potential as a woman. They're actually a tremendous gift, especially for those of us walking the path of conscious femininity.

Healing Our Shame

What stands between us viewing our cycles as our greatest blessing, rather than our most monstrous curse, is the heavy shroud of shame that ensnares them. But as renowned shame researcher and author Brené Brown teaches, shame disconnects us and, therefore, can only survive in secrecy. Once it meets empathy, it dissipates.[3]

In the SHE Retreat, we follow the arc of the Heroine's Journey over seven days. Halfway through (or just about where we are in this book right now), before we depart the depths of the underworld, we gather in a "Shame Circle." One by one, as she feels called, each woman walks into the center of the circle, takes the talking stick, and shares something she's ashamed of. Typically, women reveal deep "secrets," such as an abortion that occurred ten years ago, how cruel she is to her husband, how she still hates her body (even though she's a forty-year-old nutritionist), how her brother molested her when she was seven.

At first there are long pauses between each woman's sharing. Those who haven't yet voiced their humiliations squirm in their seats. However, several women in, something shifts. The women who have shared exude a renewed lightness and want more! The others get a whiff of this freedom and rush for their turn. They're ready to liberate themselves from their shame too.

We need to unbridle ourselves and shine light on our shame within sisterhood. Our shame shields not only the worst aspects of ourselves (demons), but also the best aspects of ourselves (daemons). Only through feeling our shame fully can we access the genius it protects. This requires a great deal of bravery, because culturally we all lack the support we need to work with such a debilitating feeling. Let's take this crucial step together.

Think back to something you feel really ashamed of. Notice the excruciating shudder that runs through your entire body as you do. Shame is one of our most physically painful emotions, so it's no wonder that it's also the root cause of so many of our addictive and abusive behaviors as we attempt to "take the edge off" its persecution.

For women, it's important to note three things:

1. Our shame arises from our Inner Critics trying to protect us from humiliation.

2. We tend to turn our aggression in on ourselves, for shame is anger directed inward. It's the root cause of our self-abuse.

3. We're most ashamed of our bodies — particularly the parts and functions of our bodies that have gone into shadow, such as our cycles, aging, postpartum depression, incontinence, organ prolapse, pelvic floor health, weight gain, etc.

The more we share our shame and partake in body-positive practices with other women, the more we can liberate ourselves from cycles of self-sabotage and free that bound-up energy for more life-enhancing creations.

Working with Your Shame

1. Name it. I once heard an interview with Brené Brown where she instructed that we silently label our sensations ("Pain. Pain. Pain!") when we feel a "shame attack" coming on. Try it. When you take this step, you effectively bring what's arising into your awareness by labeling it as a sensation. From there, you can remember that you're not a bad person; you're just *feeling* bad, momentarily. Once you can be objectively aware of something, it starts to lose its power over you.

2. Get curious about it. Where do you feel shame in your body? Look for it from the neck down. Get curious about its temperature, size, and density. Is it hot and fluttery in your chest, cold and dense in your belly, or something else entirely? Here are some examples from women in the SHE School.

- "I feel the shame in the core of my body: my stomach, my heart, my throat. The shame feels heavy, dull, and icky in my body."

- "I feel shame deep in my solar plexus as a constriction and shudder that then radiates out and draws my whole body into itself."

- "A lot of my shame lives in my throat and chest. It's also in my belly and deep in my womb too."

3. Learn your patterns. How do you react to shame? Do you move away from it by hiding, staying silent, and keeping secrets? Do you move toward it by seeking approval and to please others? Or do you move against it by being aggressive, stony, and defensive?

4. Mother yourself well. Our vulnerable children usually hold the carcasses of all our past shame. Be kind and nurturing with your Inner Little Girl when you feel a shame attack. Let her know she's safe and that you love her — no matter what.

5. Share your secrets with someone you love and trust. Your shame originated in relationship, not isolation. That's where healing needs to happen too.

6. Find the hidden fruits. Facing our shame head-on keeps us real. It allows us to confront the damage we've done in our lives and to learn from our past actions, rather than just sweep them under the rug and look the other way. Once you've named, felt, and shared your shame, write in your journal about the lessons you've learned from it. What resolves for your future actions of body, speech, and mind will you make from this clear, raw place?

SHE Cycles: Your Built-In Blueprint for Elegant Transitions

When I was in grade school, I played the piano. Every Saturday morning I went to the home of my teacher, Mrs. Cunningham, to practice my scales and tinker with whatever new pieces we were working on. I had mixed feelings about these classes. If I hadn't taken time on my own in the previous week to practice, that hour seemed to last for eons! If I *had* practiced, I felt accomplished, my fingertips floating effortlessly over the keys to serenade us. Through these conflicting experiences, I learned an important lesson: practice makes *everything* easier. Fortunately, we get regular intervals each month through our SHE Cycles to practice unconditional happiness in the face of hardships. Our cycles teach us how to withstand the inevitable difficult circumstances each month brings us — at every level. When we partner with them, we strengthen our ability to experience joy, for, ultimately, our SHE Cycles are the means through which we become our own best friends.

Each month we traverse from death to rebirth — regardless of our age. Each one of our cycles is a mini–Heroine's Journey, offering strength training for our SHEs. As our cycles ask us to oscillate our rhythms and our focus during different portions of each month, they stretch us in bite-size chunks, nudging us to slowly expand our capacity to be with the best and worst of life. They condition us to meet whatever's there. We don't need to wait to win the lottery, get sick, or stand at the deathbed of someone we most love to learn how to break open. In fact, we won't fare very well if we do. Instead, each month, when the stakes are low and no lives hang in the balance, we need to practice our "scales" by creatively engaging with the challenges and chances that each of our cycles brings. These challenges span the full spectrum of our humanity — from cramps, to work woes, to a fight with a loved one, to financial hardship, illness, and death.

When we tune into the biological rhythms that govern us, we discover that they already hold everything we need to triumph in life. Scripted into our DNA is the ancient feminine algorithm for how to transmute problems into celebrations. Our SHE Cycles serve as invaluable purification rituals. They cleanse us of what we no longer need and realign us with how we most desire to shape our futures, from within. When we ride this wave, we optimize our capability for renewal. When we fight it, we feel depleted at every level. How, then, can we stop working *against* our cycles and start working *with* them?

Even in something as mainstream and masculine as sports medicine, we see the evidence of the need to honor cycles. The secret of success for star athletes is that they embrace a new paradigm of time and energy management. To live fully, we need to act less linearly and more in rhythmic intervals. Rather than avoiding stress, we need to seek it, toggling back and forth between periods of exertion and recovery. Rather than viewing life as a marathon, we need to see it as a series of sprints. Rather than viewing rest as lazy, we need to reframe downtime as productive. Since our energy diminishes with both overuse *and* underuse, we have to continually pulse between activity and rest to be at our best.[4] This theory turns our current productivity paradigm on its head, for it posits that cycles of *both* rest *and* stress (both of which we currently judge and resist) are healthy and necessary for our evolution. If this is true for male athletes, whose cycles are far less pronounced than ours, the repercussions ring clear for women.

If we go full throttle every day of the year without a break — especially in a direction that's out of alignment with our deepest desires — we'll break down. In contrast, if we realign with our cycles, we can find a rhythm for cultivating true health, joy, and wisdom. We stretch ourselves and take risks, and then we retreat inward to recover and learn from our actions. We have built-in periods of action and reflection. In this way, we learn to play our "edge" in life.

To grow in a sane, sustainable way, you simply need to:

1. take time to get really clear about your intentions.
2. stretch out of your comfort zone for part of each month to service those intentions.
3. allow yourself a "period" of recovery.

If you follow these steps, you'll amaze yourself with who you can be and what you can accomplish with joy and ease.

The Four Seasons of Your SHE Cycle: Your Monthly Heroine's Journey

Our lives are composed of countless transitions. The moon passes through a full cycle every twenty-eight days, thirteen times a year, and a woman menstruates on average four hundred times in her life. Consequently, it makes perfect sense to reframe these recurring cycles as blueprints for moving more gracefully through our own changes.

The pattern of the four seasons, which is often used as a metaphor of life and death, lives through our monthly cycles — both through our hormones and the moon. Our cycles carry the code for working with obstacles in creative, skillful, and miraculous ways. All stages are interdependent, and creativity is only complete through the interplay of each of the seasons. Each requires that we adapt our rhythms and shape our lives around it. Now we'll explore how you can get in tune with each season of your SHE Cycle.

Below is an overview of the different facets of these cyclical patterns that we're working with each month, and over the arc of our entire lives.[5] Each stage traverses from physical to metaphysical. You can use this to better understand the multidimensionality of each of your inner and outer "seasons," and how to best align with them.

Season: Spring

Hormones: Follicular phase (lasts 7–10 days)

Moon: Waxing

Archetype: Maiden

Life stage: Childhood and adolescence

Yin/Yang: Increasing yang, decreasing yin

Hormones: Your pituitary gland sends follicle-stimulating hormone (FSH) to your ovaries, notifying them that it's time to release another egg. Simultaneously, your estrogen levels increase, thickening your uterine lining in preparation for hosting one of your eggs.

Energy level: Feel into the youthfulness of the Maiden. Notice how your physical energy keeps increasing and you feel more enthusiastic and outgoing.

Creativity: As your creativity heightens, feel within your womb what creations you're starting to nurture and grow.

Productivity: In your work life, strategize, brainstorm, network, and start new projects.

Exercise: Engage in more challenging yoga practices and workouts.

Season: Summer

Hormones: Ovulation (lasts 3–4 days)

Moon: Full

Archetype: Mother

Life stage: Adulthood

Yin/Yang: Yang

Hormones: Your FSH and luteinizing hormone levels rise, alerting a follicle to release an egg into one of your fallopian tubes, down into your
uterus. Your estrogen levels also continue to rise, still thickening your
uterine lining. Testosterone levels dip at the time of ovulation.

Energy level: You still feel energized (although you might feel a bit depleted right at ovulation).

Creativity: Like a mother, feel within your womb what creations you're
embracing.

Productivity: Since you feel the most physical and emotional stability at
this time, it's your peak time of the month. Plan your most important projects and outings for this window (business trips, dance parties
with girlfriends, project presentations, dates, sticky conversations,
vacations). Enjoy celebratory foods. Set new goals. Go full throttle.
Stretch to your edge, beyond what you think you're capable of. Live
fully and reach for your dreams!

Exercise: Go full-out with your yoga and fitness routines. Go beyond
what you think is possible for yourself, within a healthy range.

Season: Autumn

Hormones: PMS/luteal phase (lasts 10–14 days); perimenopause

Moon: Waning

Archetype: Queen

Life stage: Midadulthood

Yin/Yang: Decreasing yang, increasing yin

Hormones: The follicle from which your egg burst (your corpus luteum)
produces progesterone, which signals the uterus to keep, rather than
shed, its lining, and your estrogen levels also increase. Your period
will begin when you stop producing progesterone.

Energy level: You will feel more tired and increasingly sensitive, sus-
ceptible to darker emotions and quintessential PMS symptoms (head-
aches, moodiness, food cravings, bloating).

Creativity: Be a queen. Slow down. Look back to celebrate your harvests
from the last month and to prepare to let go of whatever didn't work out.

Productivity: Cut back on work and social commitments. Bring projects to completion. Take more time for self-care. Start turning your attention inward. Organize your home and work projects. Spend more time alone. Take more time for meditation, journaling, and sleep. Eat cleaner foods, emphasizing bitter, leafy greens to help support your liver, which is more active during this time.

Exercise: Continue to exercise, gradually dialing down your intensity. Start to shift into "recovery" mode, so that by the end of this phase you're enjoying gentle yoga and walks.

Season: Winter

Hormones: Menstruation (3–7 days)/postmenopause
Moon: New
Archetype: Crone
Life stage: Old age
Yin/Yang: Yin

Hormones: Your corpus luteum dissolves, and progesterone dips. You shed your uterine lining through your menstrual blood. Estrogen rises and then drops, informing your hypothalamus to prepare for a new cycle.

Energy level: You will feel more tired (and also relaxed) as your estrogen levels drop. You may also experience some menstrual cramps and low back pain.

Creativity: Incubate and dream your vision for the new cycle ahead. Your intuition is heightened because the connections between the right and left hemispheres of your brain are stronger now than at any other time of the month. This makes it a perfect time to meditate, journal, analyze your dreams, self-reflect, and course-correct from the past month. Turn fully into your inner wisdom. Dialogue with your SHE. Open yourself to receive her intuitive messages.

Productivity: Be the Crone. Let go and let be. Rest and hibernate.

Exercise: Practice restorative or yin yoga. Take slow walks. Move gently each day so your energy doesn't stagnate. After the first two or three days, gradually start increasing the intensity of your movement again if your body asks for it.

Through listening to our bodies' inner movements, we can't help but acknowledge that we're not "the same every day of the month," no matter what the commercials claim. Like orchids, we're very subtle, nuanced, and sensitive creatures. Rather than armoring ourselves against this exquisitely delicate aspect of our womanhood, we need to acknowledge the privilege it is to truly take care of ourselves by honoring this core dimension of our womanhood.

Uncovering the Hidden Truth of PMS

We live in a demanding world that is becoming increasingly toxic. As a result, PMS has become a modern-day, stress-induced epidemic, affecting 85 percent of menstruating women.[6] Swollen breasts and bellies. Tears without rhyme or reason. Raging words erupting from tight throats — the ones we *wish* we could take back, but can't. Ugh. Like an itch we can't stand *not* scratching, our PMS asks us to express a more authentic, and certainly *way* messier, version of ourselves.

PMS is unpredictable. It's slamming the door, or the "fuck you!" that some secret part of you really wanted to shout all month. PMS is raw. Unpredictable. Not very sexy. Not very nice at all. PMS doesn't care what other people think. PMS doesn't bother with rationalizing, taking a breath before speaking, or trying to find the middle way. PMS doesn't know how to compromise. Nor does she want to. She wants to be allowed to be wild and wrathful, however unskillful. She wants to be seen in the full glory of her power — without being judged as "hormonal."

PMS knows how to bite, fight for what she wants, and throw your inner nice girl under the bus. This dominant goody-two-shoes persona fades when the wheel of your monthly cycle dips into the dark side. In her place emerges the demanding, vulnerable you.

It's important to recognize that she lives inside *all* of us, and she needs her time in the spotlight just as much as any of our other inner selves do.

She's here to show us something more than our personalities normally allow.

This is a really the beautiful thing. PMS, like any of our dark emotions, is only an enemy when we ignore and resist her. She becomes an ally when we learn to listen to and speak her language. It's not linear and logical, like that of our conscious mind. It's metaphorical and abstract, for the symptoms serve as stewards for the *unconscious* mind. During our PMS week or days, we become different women than we are during other times of the month. Knowing this, we need to use skillful means to adjust our lives, work, and relationships accordingly.

Whatever irks us during this time is truly waving a red flag. What's in the dark comes into the light of our awareness on purpose, because each feeling points to an issue we haven't adequately resolved. These feelings have been with us, latent or less prominent, throughout every other day of the month, but now, due to our hormones, our darkness is closer to the surface. As in the fall when our psyches and immune systems are more vulnerable than they were in the summer, we need more rest and self-care now. We're more sensitive. To honor this, we need to slow down, simplify, spend more time alone, exercise in gentler ways, and expect less of ourselves. We need to reflect on the harvest from the past month. What worked well? What didn't work? What needs to be healed, let go of, or tended to more fully? Our souls want us to grow through this introspection, and they further insist upon this by giving us strong signals to help us stay or get back on track.

Every race car driver knows that the most important part of the car is the brakes. The same is true for us as women. We decelerate, rather than accelerate, into our most powerful time of the month. For this reason, we need to view PMS as a potent off-ramp into the heart of our feminine nature — the yin, *being* nexus that our menses and the new moon bring us to. From this perspective, slowing down and becoming more sensitive during these times is neither a hindrance to our success nor a sign of our weakness and incompetence. It's a privilege and a necessity.

Since yang energy always dominates — that's its nature — we need to be vigilant about cultivating equal amounts of time to prioritize yin energy. Although yin holds our feminine nature, this can be challenging if we're not trained to recognize it. Yin energy is much quieter and subtler. To find our own optimal balance between these two coessential energies, we must use our cycles as a compass to pulse out into the world for two weeks (yang), and then retreat within for the other two (yin).

"I LOVE my PMS!!" women claim when they embrace this new way of life. How well you take care of yourself each day will show up during this time. While our PMS offers a valuable training ground for being with the darker parts of our inner and outer lives, it also predicts how your perimenopause, menopause, and overall health will be later in life unless you make a change. The worse your PMS is, the more your SHE is trying to get your attention. You need to wake up and, with compassion, clearly see all the ways you're living out of alignment with your SHE's truth. Women simply can't claim true health and harmony if they ignore their monthly cycles and the roots of their imbalances.

How to Partner with Your PMS/Waning Moon Time

1. Put your PMS week on your calendar. This is your most sensitive time of the month. Mark it off in red and act accordingly! If you're married or in an intimate relationship, write it on a joint calendar. If you feel comfortable doing so, notify your family, close friends, and more intimate colleagues. Schedule yourself more lightly. Book a massage or acupuncture. Get more sleep. Meditate. Pray and open the receptive channel to your SHE. Pay attention to your dreams and intuition. Exercise in a way that's deeply nourishing — walks and yoga. Prioritize your inner world, yin time, and the lost feminine art of *being*. More gentleness and acceptance are needed at every level.

2. Listen to the messages from the dark side. Our unconscious, symbolically represented through the moon, darkness, and water, communicates with us more strongly at this time of the month (think tears and swollen body tissues). Likewise, your SHE speaks through your body and feelings. Notice the unique ways that your SHE is asking you to slow down and listen to Her. Notice signs and synchronicity. Pay close attention to challenging feelings as they arise. Traditional Chinese Medicine teaches that PMS arises from liver chi and repressed stagnant creative energy. Explore ways that you're ignoring or stifling your creativity. All of these hold the key to staying positively engaged throughout this period of "destruction." For help with supporting your liver, please see part 2 of *The Way of the Woman*.

3. Find the medicine in the symptom. Make a list of all the ways that you experience PMS — and what you get irritated and upset by during this time. Don't act on these insights quite yet. The action time will come in the two weeks after your period. For now, just use this time to listen and discern. Next to each symptom, write down what you believe its medicine is. What does each of these irritants have to teach you? There are more tools for this below.

4. Create a new plan for the month ahead. Based on what you are noticing, what shifts can you make in the month ahead? How can you reduce stress (the main cause of PMS) and take better care of your body? How can you honor your feelings? Which feelings do you believe it's not okay for you to express? To whom do you need to speak your truth and build better boundaries? What do you need to let go of? In what ways do you long to express your creative passions?

5. Mother yourself well. As women, we have the power to listen, learn, revamp, and grow each and every month. Some months will be more stressful than others. That's okay. Remember, this isn't about being perfect. It's about slowing down enough to listen to our bodies and our SHEs. Be a good mother to yourself — embrace your process with un-conditional love. Connect with your Inner Little Girl. Ask yourself: What are my basic needs here? What helps me to feel whole and connected?

6. Rock your sacred NO. Say "no" *frequently* — way more often than feels comfortable. Before expending your precious creative energy on a project, check in with your body. If you're not a full-bodied "hell YES!" then you're a no. Ask yourself: Where am I caught in pleasing others? What am I saying yes to that really doesn't feel good? Where am I trying to compete or live up to someone else's standards of success? What can I say no to? How can I do less here?

Working with Strong Feelings

If we want to really get to know happiness and joy, we need to become intimate with their opposites. The darker sides of our cycles (PMS, fall/winter, waning/new moon) give us ample opportunity to do so. In meeting all of our feelings with steadfast love and attention, we learn first-hand that whatever is part of our human condition is part of our path to wholeness. We're not looking to eradicate our afflictive feelings, because their absence won't indicate our success. We're learning to cultivate emotional maturity by sourcing innovative ways for working with whatever is arising. This attitude of friendly, curious willingness emancipates our demons, allowing them to reveal to us fresh ways for engaging with conflict.

Get interested if something feels difficult to you, because all of our feelings carry information. They signal that there's an unmet need you must attend to. Just as the cries of babies signal to parents that they're hungry, your anger, anxiety, doubt, fear, and sadness warn you that something's amiss. You need to use your meditation practice, especially during your vulnerable times of each month, to remind yourself to view your dark feelings (especially the ones that you have the most resistance to) as invaluable messengers of your SHE's guidance, rather than as enemies.

Here's a technique for working with strong feelings of affliction. Let's try it now, together.

The RAIN Practice

Locate in your awareness something right now that feels unsatisfactory. Perhaps it's a sensation in your body, an emotion, a recurring thought. It could be a sound in your environment, or that you're too hot or cold. If you can't find one thing right now that feels unpleasant, think back to a time earlier today. Got it?

Recognition: Notice that a feeling is arising and name it for yourself (e.g., "I feel angry"). Note that language is important here. Rather than saying "I'm angry" and identifying with the anger, say "I feel angry" so you can see it as a temporary experience that isn't forever "you." I'll say it again: recognition opens the doorway to release.

Acceptance: Allow that sensation to be here. Cultivate an environment of compassion and physically *feel* whatever is arising *from your heart.* Can you even accept your resistance to it?

Investigation: Get curious about the sensation, like a mother looking intently at her infant daughter's face to read whether she's hungry, tired, or needs a change of diapers. Where is it in your body, exactly? What are its specific characteristics? Does it have a color? Temperature? Texture and density?

Nonidentification: When a mother holds her child, allowing her to cry (without smothering, controlling, or trying to manipulate her experience), her daughter feels safe to be just as she is. Can you offer this to yourself when you're uncomfortable? Don't get enmeshed in how to "fix" the discomfort. Know that the discomfort is not "you." It's a fleeting experience. The more you allow the discomfort to be here, just as it is, the more effortlessly it can flow and transform into something else. Stay out of the story and in your body. Relax around the intensity and allow the feeling to flow, shift, and change. Every feeling has a lifespan of only about ninety seconds when we don't interfere with it. Remind yourself, "This too shall pass."

Suffering only arises when our preferred reality doesn't line up with actual reality. The pain of life, and of our cycles, is real, but our suffering is optional. Let's dig a little deeper and explore how to apply these practices with one of our most universally disowned feelings — anger.

Accessing Your Anger

Feminine anger is both a personal and a collective taboo. During PMS it bubbles and erupts like a volcano, making it a potent time to transmute it. We all relate to anger in one of two ways:

1. **We stuff it and deny our needs.** This imploded anger becomes toxic shame and resentment. It's the root of self-violence,

self-sabotage, and addiction. We're afraid to get angry with others, so we turn it all inward, onto ourselves.

2. **We project it onto others.** We scream at our kids, curse in traffic, take it out on our dog, snap at the bank clerk, or shame our spouses.

In either case, the anger isn't clean. Both approaches are equally painful. Since there's no "I" in it, it's disowned. As little girls we're taught that it's not okay to be angry, yet we cannot incarnate our power without reclaiming our wrath. We *need* our anger and its fiery clarity to love fiercely, set clear boundaries, and protect those we love from danger. Anger is valuable when it speaks what it sees and creates change rather than destroys. Just like all of our feelings, anger carries a message. Harriet Lerner, PhD, and author of *The Dance of Anger*, shares, "Just as physical pain tells us to take our hand off the hot stove, the pain of our anger preserves the very integrity of our self."[7]

Years, and even decades, of being disconnected from our anger can lead to all sorts of problems:

Liver congestion: According to Traditional Chinese Medicine, the liver is the storehouse of anger.

Fatigue and depression: Anger is a life force, and when we do not allow it to flow freely, we stagnate.

Painful cycles and menopause: These are also symptoms of liver congestion.

Relationships destroyed by resentment or abuse: These occur when we didn't say what we needed to say, or we did say it, but in a harmful way.

Diving Deeper into Your Anger

To help you extract the wisdom from your anger, answer the following questions, adapted from Harriet Lerner's book *The Dance of Anger*, in your journal:

1. What am I really angry about?
2. What's the real underlying issue here?

3. How does this mirror a familiar, unresolved situation from my child-hood?
4. What's my position?
5. What are my needs here?
6. What's mine to own and what isn't?
7. What's my desired outcome? How can I take the high road without being a doormat?
8. Where do I need to stand firm and where do I need to compromise and draw a boundary?[8]

Additional Practices

1. Ask yourself: Can I view this irritation as my path? This turns it from an enemy into a doorway.
2. Ventilate your irritations. Write down everything that's irking you. Then ceremoniously rip or burn the list.
3. Have a conscious temper tantrum. Turn on some music and, for a song that lasts at least two minutes, let the energy move through you without inhibition. Yell, curse, stomp your feet. Get it out.
4. Remember that when you're angry, it's because you care about something deeply. Get in touch with your heart and see what's needing your protection.

Through aligning your life around your SHE Cycles and gaining the wise-woman skills you need to decipher your SHE's secret callings hidden inside your PMS, you can use this tumultuous time to fuel your grandest life vision. Stop running from the darkness that your cycles bring. Instead, channel their mysterious power and creativity into the hardest places in your life. Capture the magic that lives inside you right now and that is your birthright as a woman.

Journaling Questions

- What is your physical and emotional history with your creative organs? Describe your relationship to them, since your adolescence. Do you notice any themes or recurring messages?
- Which phase of our four-part cycle is easiest for you to embrace? Which is the most challenging? What are the driving behaviors and beliefs behind this imbalance? What repercussions does this have in your life?
- What is your relationship to anger? How do you usually express it? Does your response impact what you discovered in the previous two reflections?

Chapter 8

Meditating
on Your Mortality

When we menstruate there has been a death.
A child will not be born. But there is a possibility of new spiritual life....
If we don't take time to respect these mysteries, we feel a terrific tension.

— Marion Woodman, *Conscious Femininity*

As part of my "First Thought" practice to enter the day with a sacred view, each morning before I get out of bed, I recite to myself the "Four Mind Changings" from Tibetan Buddhism.[1] The second of these is: "Everything is impermanent. This ephemeral existence is not to be wasted. Everyone who is born will die. My death is certain, the exact time is unknown. Knowing this, what is most important?"[2]

Let's wake up each day with gratitude that we have another day to live and with the remembrance that it could be our last. One day, maybe today or tomorrow or twenty years from now, everything that seems so solid and secure can, and will, fall away.

Depending on our family and religious backgrounds, we may have been raised to fear death. However, death isn't the end of life. It's the opening to the other side of it. Death enhances life when we live with it in the forefront of our minds.

How can we learn to live with the truth that every day we're getting closer to our final exhale? If we take the ten-thousand-foot view of *all* the stages of our SHE Cycles, we see a way to do this. If we practice dying each month, we'll live as many moments as we can with the recognition of life's preciousness. Through our SHE Cycles, we create the lives of our dreams in order to die without regrets. Each month's dip into death and resurrection, when we partner with them consciously, primes us for the greatest rite of passage of all — death.

Your Monthly Death:
The New Moon and the First Day of Your Cycle

The best place to begin working with this new paradigm is on the first day of your cycle, or on the first day of the new moon if you don't have your cycle. If you are only following the moon, you won't need to make as many physical adjustments as I discuss in this section because you aren't bleeding, but during those times you should still prioritize rest, being over doing, visioning, and tuning into intuition.

Also, for optimal health, it's ideal for women to menstruate on the new moon, thus honoring both "rest points" at the same time. However, most of us are out of synch with this rhythm. That's okay, so be careful not to get caught up in "fixing" or "perfecting" your cycles. Doing so will lead you away from the point of all this! If the lunar cycle doesn't line up with your menstruation, like one hand patting your head while another rubs your belly, participate in both of these cycles. Prioritize physically resting on the first days of your cycle, but also acknowledge the letting go time of the new moon.

For women, the first day of the cycle is by far *the most important day of the month*. It's the still point — the day of complete yin and potentiated rest and recovery. When you participate in the replenishing energy that's available on this day, you're supercharged. Your tired body and mind can rejuvenate far more easily at this time than they can on other days of the month, because you're working *with* the energy that's already present, rather than against it.

Most of us have been raised to think that it's weak or simply not necessary to take time off during our periods, or to think that we don't need special attention on these days. Instead we feel we need to prove we can "take it like a man." However, if we resist and deny this energy, our batteries will drain out more quickly, both on that day and during the rest of the month. We each must investigate our own judgments, prejudices, and resistances to resting, bleeding, and allowing our bodies to renew each month.

While *rest* is often treated like a four-letter curse in our society, its value is priceless. I once heard Madonna note during an interview that the most life-altering spiritual practice she ever engaged in was to practice *savasana* (the corpse pose) for thirty minutes a day. A bona fide overachiever, she knew that the medicine she needed most — letting go, opening, and being — resided in the practice of feigning death and doing absolutely nothing. Likewise, Taoist traditions teach that the most profound practice is simply to open ourselves and become receptive to the universal creative energy that's always available to us. Reclaiming rest as a priority in our daily, weekly, monthly, seasonal, and yearly rhythms stands as the most profound spiritual practice that we can integrate into our lives.

The first step toward honoring your cycle is to start tracking it — just as we did with our PMS. Become conscious of when the first day of your cycle and the new moon are, and put those dates on your calendar. To the degree that you feel comfortable, communicate to colleagues and loved ones that this is the first day of your SHE Cycle. Explain that the more you can rest and recharge on that day, the more you can be of service on all other days of the month.

Next, build your schedule around your cycle. If possible, block off the first day to have it completely to yourself. Don't schedule meetings, work trips, workshops, deadlines, parties, or phone calls. Nothing. Consider taking a sick day, trading a day off for working on a weekend, or, if you are home with small children, swapping childcare with a friend.

If you can't take the first day of your cycle off, but you can take the second or third day off, go for it. And of course, if the work or travel opportunity falls only during your cycle, you don't have to say no to it. The most important thing is to stop and ask yourself what you need, and then work with your inner selves (especially your Inner Little Girl) so your decision reflects every part of you.

For those months when you can't take the day off, your inner attitude is the most important thing. Focus on gentleness and rest. Even if you have a full day of work or childcare, bring your hot water bottle with you and rest it on your belly when you're at your desk. Wear a super-comfy outfit. Bring a cozy shawl or blanket to wrap around you. Carry a thermos of hot raspberry leaf tea. Pack your own lunch, like a hot soup or stew and a salad or steamed vegetables, and have a quiet date with yourself. Do the absolute minimum amount of work that you can to get by. Accept that this is not your most "on" day, and don't push it.

Immerse yourself in the mindset of "There's nothing else for me to do right now but rest." Get takeout or delivery. Put your feet up. Snuggle on the couch. On this day, you want to get as still and quiet as possible. This is part of your SHE space, your time to prioritize being instead of doing. Through this, you open a portal to your Inner SHE — your intuition — to receive valuable visions and guidance for the month ahead.

Here are more specific suggestions for you to try. Remember that none of these are set in stone. See what works for you, and customize rituals for your own cycle.

What to Do on the First Few Days of Your Cycle

- Pay attention to your dreams. Ask specific questions before you go to sleep. Then, instead of jumping out of bed in the morning, linger for a while. Contemplate your dreams. Write them down. While they are still fresh in your psyche, start to digest them.
- Sleep as long as you need to, or take a nap midday.
- Stay in silence as much as possible.
- Meditate.
- Walk in nature.
- Practice yin and/or restorative yoga.
- Turn off your phone and computer. Unplug!
- Eat simply and cleanly — cut out sugar, caffeine, alcohol, refined foods, and common allergens like gluten and dairy, to help keep your mind clear.

- Draw, collage, or paint.
- Visualize your desired life for the new cycle ahead.
- Write in your journal (see recommended reflection questions later on in this chapter).
- Spend some time in the company of other trusted women. Share your visions. Receive feedback and reflection. Be witnessed in your depths.
- Use reusable organic cotton pads or a menstrual cup rather than synthetic tampons and pads. This helps to deepen your intimacy with your body and her cycles, while keeping your most sacred parts safe from toxins. Many women who have gone through my programs also note that their PMS diminishes through embracing this one simple step.
- Create your own SHE Cycle rituals. Choose a few things that you'll do during every cycle to remind yourself of this sacred pause. Some of the women in our community dress in red, cook big pots of soup, have partners bring home takeout for dinner, stay in their pajamas all day, or burn red candles on their altars.

What Not to Do on the First Day of Your Cycle

- Have wild sex (or even have sex at all). See what it's like to keep your body for yourself on this day.
- Go out drinking and dancing.
- Take a hot bath or sauna. This is a protocol from Ayurveda and Traditional Chinese Medicine. Our menstrual blood is already "hot," and our bodies are trying to "cool off" through our bleeding, so it's best not to add more heat.
- Go to the gym or do any sort of vigorous yoga or exercise. Our wombs are bigger and heavier now than they are at other times of the month. Therefore, it's best not to strain them through a lot of jumping around. I do think it's important to move on these days — but that means a gentle walk outside and some yin and/or restorative yoga. Use this day as a time to let go of your more intensive exercise routines.

- Spend the day on the Internet. Go offline. Turn away from the voices and opinions of others so you can tune in to the rhythms of nature and your own inner wisdom.
- Clean the house. I hear from some women that they love to clean house on these days, but I advocate that, at least on your first day, you don't do any chores. Being is hard for us at this time in history. Practice giving yourself at least one day a month to have no agenda and no to-do list to complete.
- Errands. Again, remain in rest-and-receiving mode. This is a great time to practice asking for help rather than being the responsible superwoman who does it all.
- Cook for the whole family. Instead, have your partner make dinner or bring home takeout. Have something delivered or cook a big pot of soup earlier in the month, freeze it, and heat up the leftovers. Eat healthy, wholesome foods that you don't have to cook!

It takes time and persistent dedication to design our lives around our cycles. Each month we can tinker with these practices, deepen, and learn. Choose one or two new ones to experiment with. Once those feel natural, choose one or two more. I've been working with this for over a decade, and still there are some months when it's not possible for me to take time off during my cycle. We're not going for rigid perfection here; we're dancing with an ideal. A little goes a long way. Each month will look how it needs to look. As always, allow your own experience to guide you and remember the concept of "good enough." When you start to feel the positive effects of living like this, your attraction to feeling good will guide you further.

Period Power: Channeling the Red-Robed Goddess

Native American traditions referred to menstruating women as "being on their moon." It was a time when women gathered together, away from their children and the men, in a Moon Lodge to cleanse, dream, and rest.

Women, these ancients believed, didn't have to go on vision quests like their men did. They could access their insight through the visions that came through their menses. These elders wove into the fabric of their communities what we forgot long ago: Each cycle purifies us and allows us to create life anew. These mini-deaths are times to pause, reflect, and realign to see if we're creating the legacies that we want to leave behind. Through this, menses can be a time of deep creativity and conscious renewal that most of us overlook and misunderstand. They give us the space to dig into raw potentiality to source new solutions to our problems. If we don't use the energy of our wombs to grow a baby, we can instead harness that life-giving power to create a better life and world.

If we remember how to participate in this deep, internal mystery that each of us is born with, then when we come to our bigger initiations, we can trust that we have the inner resources and clear seeing we need to help us move through life with wisdom and grace. Our cycles train us to stay rooted in our inner ground in the midst of life's greatest storms. First we practice this for ourselves, and eventually we're able to offer it as a gift and service to our loved ones and communities. In order to evolve as a species, we *need* the emergent wisdom from our cycles to be made conscious. As women, this is one of the most valuable contributions we can offer the world.

The Magic of Moon Blood

Holy places are dark places.... Holy wisdom is not clear
and thin like water, but thick and dark like blood.

— C. S. Lewis, *Till We Have Faces*

We're all born in the water of the womb, and water has long been the domain of the Goddess. It symbolizes the source of life and is a vehicle for death and resurrection. This holy water moves through us each month in the stream of menstrual blood.

In ancient goddess cultures, the magical elixir of creation was thought to reside in this menstrual blood, or Moon Blood (MB). Called "the Holy Blood of Life," it was viewed as the sustenance of the Divine Mother. A woman's womb was seen as the life-giving vessel, and the monthly cleansing and purification of this chalice was her menstruation. Her cycles were the initiations through which she deepened her relationship to the mystery of the Sacred Feminine.

Relating to our MB in a positive way helps us to feel a renewed sense of respect and awe for our magical female bodies. It serves as a mystical bridge between our human selves and the Divine Mother. When our MB flows, our SHEs speak more strongly to us. The more attention you pay to your MB, the more it will reflect back your current state of health and happiness each month. Some of the first questions a skilled Traditional Chinese Medicine doctor will ask you are: How is your cycle? What does your menstrual blood look like? The more we pay attention to our MB's color, texture, and flow, the more we can stay aware of deeper physical, emotional, and spiritual shifts transpiring within us.

This is how some women in our community now describe their healed relationships with their MB:

> "About a year ago I began a deep transformation in my relationship with my blood. I never really found my blood 'appealing'/'interesting' or anything really positive, 'just blood.'...Now I actually found it beautiful."

> "It has become a bridge, a form of dialogue with my body. I like to use reusable cotton pads just to keep this special bond conscious."

> "My cycle just returned after a one-year absence. Today I feel as though I am becoming a woman perhaps for the first time in my life. Today I am not denying any part of myself."

> "My SHE is telling me that something deeper is awakening inside — a rebirth, new life — and I feel that through my bleeding. It is not painful. It feels healing and restoring rather than draining. My SHE is literally singing now whereas before I started this work SHE was stone cold and barely breathing."

Journal Reflections for Your SHE Cycle

- What judgment and prejudices do you have about your cycle?
- What was your menarche like? Recall all the details and feelings around your first period. Visit the practices for working with shame in the previous chapter, if needed.
- What rituals do you want to employ to honor your SHE Cycle this month?
- What are you releasing from this past month? What needs to be shed, released, and allowed to die?
- What are you longing to create and give birth to in the month ahead? What seeds are you planting for dreams and visions for next month's cycle?
- What are you not seeing that wants to be seen?

Perimenopause:
Preparing for Your True Wisdom Initiation

After many years of conscious cycling, we discover that we evolve through reduction and re-creation during our monthly periods. All seems to be going well until we fall into one of the biggest black holes in women's health: perimenopause. This potent phase often goes unrecognized by women, despite its rather blaring symptoms. Most of us don't even *know* what perimenopause is! Once again, our distance from the truth leaves us feeling alone and fatally flawed. But as the big sister of PMS, perimenopause is an incredibly potent initiation for *all* women, whether you're experiencing it now, it's already past for you, or it's something you need to start preparing for.

Perimenopause stands as the transition between menstruation and menopause. Technically, menopause lasts only one day — the one that falls exactly twelve months after your last menses. Everything *after* that day is considered to be postmenopause, and everything before that day, but after your cycles become more irregular, is considered to be *peri*menopause. According to the National Institute on Aging, the average age for menopause in women in developed countries is fifty-one. Perimenopause starts, on average, anywhere between the ages of thirty-five and forty-two, and can last for several years.[3] There are also many cases of surgically induced menopause, which can happen at any age and bypasses perimenopause because it comes on so suddenly.

In general, perimenopause's larger purpose is not to antagonize us, but to best prepare us to live the last season of our lives with authenticity. This time is now being marked by a new, emergent archetype of the Queen, for she represents the sagacity a woman has amassed not only from her motherhood phase, but also from all of her previous life's experiences. With the lifespan of women continually increasing, the Queen steps in to serve as the archetypal bridge between Mother and Crone during the widening gap between middle and old age.

How do we recognize perimenopause? Hot flashes, irregular cycles, weight gain, and an intensification of PMS symptoms. Dr. Christiane Northrup describes it as PMS multiplied by *ten*.[4]

As with our monthly cycles, perimenopause differs a lot from woman to woman. How it impacts you is tied into the answers to some of the following questions:

- How old was your mother when she went through menopause?
- What kind of menopause did she have?
- What is your diet like?
- Do you get enough pleasurable movement?
- What is your stress level?
- Are you in fulfilling relationships?
- Do you have any past trauma that you haven't faced?
- Do you feel creatively expressed?
- Have you accepted the truth that you're aging?
- Do you enjoy your work?
- Are you getting enough sleep?
- Are you speaking your truth?
- Are there any areas of your life where you're not taking full ownership?

From a larger, spiritual perspective, perimenopause is a finale to PMS. It's a midlife cleansing of rage and resentment, releasing previously blocked creative expression through its heat. The physical discomfort and rage that arise are simply undigested emotions surfacing from our unconscious, into the light of our loving awareness. When we judge and resist our rage, it only roars louder: "I am your power!"

To align the final chapters of our lives fully with our SHEs, we will need to direct this inner fire to fuel the very tough changes that we may need to make. The edges of the path get sharper and the stakes get higher the older we get, for our bodies and SHEs are less tolerant of our abuse and neglect than they were when we were younger. Perimenopause is an ally, for it calls us to do our work and to clean up any unfinished business of the past. That's the only way we can call in the love, joy, and abundance that we are destined for in the final chapters of our lives.

To embrace this portal into Queenhood, let's be honest about all the things we fear and resist about it. We're *all* aging. Perimenopause just makes it more apparent that we're on the waning end of life's crescent.

Here are some fears about aging that perimenopausal women in our community shared:

"I fear that I will be less juicy, less vibrant, less alive."

"I'm afraid of weight gain and the loss of my woman-hood."

"I feel like I will be less desirable or that I have no value."

"I fear that I will lose my vitality. I am already slowing down in movement due to joint sensitivities, less energy, feeling down on myself, etc."

"I'm afraid of death and dying. I'm worried I will be less desirable. I'm sad about losing womanhood during this time."

Explore Your Relationship to Aging

Write down your own fears and beliefs about aging. Don't censor yourself. Be honest. Take a full inventory.

- How did your mother work with her own aging process?
- What positive female role models do you have for aging gracefully?
- How do you want to age?

The Metamorphosis of Menopause

A woman's postmenopausal phase offers her the chance to become more and more intimate with her mortality, making the final quarter (or perhaps half) of her life a period of completion. Now, rather than shedding her creations each month, she contains all of her energy inside of her. She moves into the seat of the elder through holding this wisdom in her body and using it to continue to tend to any unfinished business before her final transition; to enjoy the world, just as it is; and to serve her community through her knowledge.

Sadly, there aren't many role models of women who are embracing their aging process in this way, although some wonderful examples include Helen Mirren, Meryl Streep, Betty White, Jane Fonda, Gloria Steinem, Maya Angelou, and Oprah Winfrey. We live in a world where external, youthful feminine beauty is valued over feminine wisdom. However, we truly are like fine wines. We grow richer and more valuable with age, but only when we devote ourselves to doing our inner work. Otherwise we stay trapped as insecure little girls inside aging bodies!

In ancient goddess cultures, many of the shamans, witches, and medicine women — or powerful community healers — were originally postmenopausal women. These are the elders who hold real wisdom, because a woman inhabits her fullest power after menopause. She has more psychic energy available to her. She's no longer governed so strongly by her emotions, nor is she fixated on her family and career. She trusts the cycles of life and her ability to navigate them. She's less insecure and no longer interested in pleasing others or gaining their approval. She's focused on answering life's most important questions: How well have I lived and loved? How can my presence serve and heal others?

Like our periods, menopause is a time for us to rest, pause, and gain spiritual insight. The less experience we have with sitting still with our darkness when we're younger, the harder it will be later in life. Regardless of age, this is still an essential skill to cultivate.

In her book *The Wisdom of Menopause*, Dr. Christiane Northrup points out that our menopause today is very different from that of our mothers and grandmothers. A hundred years ago, most women didn't live long enough to even go through perimenopause — much less menopause. We're all pioneers in rewriting the significance of our "new middle age."[5]

Traditional Chinese Medicine calls menopause our "second spring," for when we approach menopause, we're preparing to give birth to the happiest, most honest version of ourselves we've ever known. Many women are shown to have their creative peaks at the age of fifty, and these peaks often last twenty-five to thirty years.[6] If we've been ignoring our own needs or creative passions at the expense of caring for others, we reach a place where we can no longer tolerate that.

Menopause is a time that asks women to strike a new balance between being and doing, enacting the youthful energy to nurture new hobbies, businesses, and self-identities while also drawing upon the elder energy to practice simply being. In all cases, postmenopause asks each woman to stop and reevaluate her life. Many women experience dissolution at this time. Their marriages fall apart, they endure the death or ailment of a spouse or parent, or they change careers. It's not an option to keep living in the same way. As women experience menopause, they must take the time and get the support necessary to process whatever arises in welcoming and adapting to this new life season.

Musing on Menopause

As you prepare yourself for menopause or support yourself through it, consider the answers to these essential questions:

- What are you not saying that needs to be said? What unmet needs are you still tolerating?
- What do you still not accept about yourself?
- How fulfilled do you feel in these areas: creativity, health, relationship, finances, spirituality?
- Where are some better boundaries needed?
- What wisdom do you carry that you're not fully owning and offering to others?
- What do you feel you *must* do before you die, and what's a small step you can take today toward fulfilling that?

The Crone Is Back,
and She's Not Just for Our Golden Years

Whatever age we are right now, we need to call upon the long-lost goddess of aging — the Crone — to help us embrace our own impermanence. What do you feel in your body and envision in your mind when you hear this word *crone*? Do you see a shriveled old woman? A powerful sorceress? Do you feel a cringe in your chest? Or something else?

Whenever I teach about the Crone, most women have a strong reaction to her. "Come on! Can't we find another word here?" they lament, "like Queen, or something more...empowering?"

My response is always: NO! Because you can't get any more powerful than the Crone. She's the cumulative apex of our womanhood, conjoining all of our hard-earned life wisdom into an archetype that is larger than any of us.

Archetypes are like energetic holograms, holding evolutionary patterns of unfolding that transcend culture, time, and space. Asking to change an archetype is like asking to change the ocean's tides. *It's simply not up to us.* The force is far too great, and we are too small. You cannot change the name of the Crone, but you can channel her power, and her wisdom.

The Crone is an archetype that has been ostracized and forgotten. She's been pushed into the cellars of our collective unconscious. If a woman is old, we think she's worthless. If she's wrinkled, she's invisible. Only the Maiden — voluptuous, cream-skinned, thick-haired — is powerful in our view. But the Maiden's power is only skin deep. She does not *yet* know how to love herself. She does not *yet* know how to express her full truth. She does not *yet* know how to access those parts of herself that are indestructible — untouched by birth, old age, sickness, and death. Only the Crone can do this.

The Patriarchy fears the Crone, for she represents a completely different kind of power than we see alive in the world today. Her power is mysterious, internal, intuitive, and fierce. It's rare to find a Crone now, but every community needs at least one.

This original meaning of the Crone was a very positive one: "She has nothing to lose. Who she is cannot be taken away from her. She has no investment in ego.... She's a perfect mirror for a person."[7] The modern dictionary, however, defines *crone* as "an old woman who is thin and ugly."[8]

Somewhere along the way, along with the repression of goddess culture and the shaming of women's bodies and cycles, the concept of the Crone was erroneously redefined — placing it in the most negative of lights. Knowing this, the act of true empowerment here is not to buy into this modern, patriarchal definition by rejecting it — and therefore accepting it. Real power comes through reappropriation.

Who Is the Crone, Really? And Why Do We Need Her?

The Maiden creates new life, the Mother sustains it, and the Crone dissolves it. She doesn't care what anyone thinks of her. She doesn't try to placate, assuage, or please. She says what she means and means what she says. The Crone is the one whom we can call upon when we feel insecure and unsure, when we feel afraid that our own truth will alienate us by causing others to criticize or condemn. Her only desire is to be herself, in every situation. In fact, she's the perfect mirror in any situation, because she carries no agenda other than delivering the truth. She likes to cackle and poke fun. She enjoys being a trickster and causing a spectacle. She never settles for anything other than the truth.

The Crone speaks like a whip. Her words come in a single crack, with no reverberating pain: *SLAP!*

The Crone's wisdom is hard earned. Through her suffering she has come to know herself. She has traveled over and over into the darkness. She knows that comfort comes only through discomfort, and that liberation can come only from within.

The Crone lives in the woods, or at the edge of villages. Those who are on the brink of life and death — birthing mothers, diseased elders, brokenhearted warriors — seek her out. The Crone can see every situation for exactly what it is. She can deliver the medicine, even if it burns or causes more suffering before the healing can set in.

Crones do not live outside of us; they live within us. An eighty-year-old still may not be a Crone; a twenty-five-year-old may be deeply in touch with her. Our Inner Crones reflect our relationships to our inner worlds. A rich inner life cultivates wisdom and courage. The Crone is the gatekeeper of these. Women of all ages need access to the Crone, particularly in times when we are afraid to speak what's on our minds, can't find our truth, or can't feel our power. If we have a hard time making a decision, we need to call on her.

She exists in quiet moments. She's the voice of clarity that rings through the confusion when we turn our attention inward and listen. Her voice gets stronger and louder the more we trust and confide in her. Bring your Inner Crone into the areas of your life that need her most.

The Crone is here with us now, in our darkest moments before the dawn of our Heroine's Journey. She's reminding us that there's nothing more for us to do.

Our work is done, for now. Our time down here is almost complete. It's time to simply rest in the pregnant void of the underworld. Before moving on, please spend some time alone in the dark. Light a candle in your sacred space. Remain still and silent. Listen. Be fed by the fertile darkness. Our surrender will signal the One who will come to light the way for our transfiguration.

Journaling Questions

- What is your relationship to death? How has it visited you in your life so far? What scares you about it? What have you learned from it?

- Do you rest enough? In what ways do you resist it? What's hard, or delicious, about sitting still?

- How do you envision yourself at the end of your life? What kind of woman do you want to be? Does she have any wisdom to share with you now?

- What areas of your life could benefit from the wisdom of your Inner Crone?

Part III

The Initiation

When you do something, you should burn yourself completely,
like a good bonfire, leaving no trace of yourself.

— Suzuki Roshi, in *Enter the Heart of the Fire*
by Mary E. Giles and Kathryn Hohlwein

The Golden Dakini

St. Benedict's Monastery, Snowmass, Colorado; December 17, 2011

Several months after I told Sofia about my first apparition of Mary Magdalene, and after many baby steps of opening up to Her divine communication each day, I took my first major leap in forging my own spiritual path and trusting Mary's guidance. She told me to visit a place I'd never been before: a Benedictine monastery in Snowmass, Colorado.

I had been practicing Buddhism for just over a decade at that point, and that visit signified my first step toward integrating the Catholic roots I had abandoned in my teens. My intention for the retreat was to commune with Mary more deeply and to get closer to the heart of why She had returned into my life.

During my weeklong, solitary retreat, I further trusted myself by crafting my own schedule in a way that honored both my path *and* the retreat center's lineage: I attended Mass with the monks in the early mornings, meditated throughout the day, took walks in the snowy silence, practiced yoga in the late afternoons, and commenced "Centering Prayer," a form of devotional inner listening taught by the monastery's former head abbot, Father Thomas Keating.

I spent most of my time alone, save daily Mass, when I sat alongside the twelve monks who lived at the monastery. Although the surroundings looked very masculine on the surface, their spirited liturgies and the stained glass above the altar allowed me to feel Mary's presence very strongly. I sensed that, underneath everything, there shimmered the soft, soothing Sacred Feminine, and that somehow my presence there strengthened that. But I still wasn't yet clear about exactly why Mary had led me there.

On my fourth day, in the pregnant epicenter of my retreat, right about when things always get really hard before they get better, I woke up with a feeling of massive anxiety and stuck-ness in my solar plexus. This had been a common, recurring feeling throughout my life, often leading me to binge and purge, and that day I felt its ominous power. It seemed to muddy everything — my work, relationships, health, finances, body image, and self-esteem. As the intensity in my core only increased as the day went on, I turned to the practice of one of my teachers, Lama Tsultrim Allione, to transmute that demon into a daemon.

During the first step of this practice, which she calls "Feeding Your Demons," I closed my eyes and felt the thick intensity in my middle. I noted its essential qualities: heavy, wide, like a big rectangle. I looked more closely for additional details: red, kind of a rusty red, cold. Actually, a brick. I then personified the brick, seeing it sitting across from me, and I listened to what it wanted and needed from me: love. As I fed the brick demon the nectar of my love, gradually its denseness started to shift and shine. Then it dissolved into a liquid heap on the floor, out of which emerged a woman. A dancing woman. A golden, dancing woman. A golden, dancing Dakini. From my inner impasse emerged flow. Beauty. Grace Herself.

"What message do you have for me?" I asked this golden ally. I paused and listened, crinkling my nose and forehead, and let my lips curl into a sly smile as I heard her response.

She replied, "I am you and you are me. You are powerful beyond your wildest comprehension. I'll show you the way."

Three days later, I dug deep, summoning the will to make it through the last yoga practice of my weeklong solitary retreat. I was ready to go home. It was twilight on the eve before my favorite day of the year — the winter solstice — so even though it was only five o'clock, the sky had already swallowed everything in black, save Venus, who glittered a blue blessing over the snowy mountain valley beyond my picture window. The finale of the week left a lot to delight in, and I was ready to celebrate. Even though I usually don't practice yoga to music, I looked through iTunes, searching for the right music to inspire me.

Om Mane Padme Hum. Om Mane Padme Hum.

This ancient Tibetan chant means "The jewel of the lotus flower [the ancient symbol of awakening in Buddhism] lives within." Like a playful cat ready to pounce, the chant slipped into the room and then into me. My palms spread on the mat. Breath ballooned my thighs and belly. Each lunge of my legs and arch of my back made my body more fully mine. Rising up to stand at the top of my yoga mat, my arms began to wave, unscripted and spontaneously, like magic wands through the cool air of the hermitage, casting long shadows in the candlelight.

On my altar, Mary overlooked my practice, which had by then become an unchoreographed dance. Seeming to smile back at me, She had been my steady companion and guide all week. That night, no longer strangers, we moved together, one heart, one body, this breath, until a golden radiance began to ripple out of each of my movements — into my breasts, hips, and the spread of each of my toes. My fingertips pranced in ancient *mudras*, ritual gestures and energetic seals that I had never before learned yet now knew so well. I wasn't "doing" yoga; yoga was "doing" *me*.

Tears, like luminescent war paint, glistened on my cheeks. Laughter spilled from my throat into the silent room. For how hard everything always seemed and for how good it had really been all along. At myself for forgetting to get the joke, and for being the brunt of it. Laughter at the delight of being free from my past. Free from my story. Free from my suffering. Free from myself. Free.

Before then, I had known *samadhi*, a Buddhist term that represents the joy that arises from the realization of nondual consciousness, like the monks did: a still, silent, empty euphoria. But that night, I knew it as only a woman could, through the curves of my body, up the ecstasy of my snaking spine. A pink blessing flowed out from my heart like warm honey into the night. In that moment I knew I had not been guided there to get something from the monks, but to bless them with this dance. I danced also for my family, my beloved, and my students. I danced for my challenges and for every moment that had brought me there. I danced for and with my teacher, Sofia, because she was the one who taught me the dance. I danced in awe for the fruits of many years, lifetimes even, of practice that graced me in that moment.

I danced as and for my True Self. I *was* the Golden Dakini. Dripping with the ambrosia of goodness and all things deliciously alive, my body leapt and twisted into spontaneous, ancient shapes of beauty. The consort to nothingness, I danced in rapturous communion with the Sacred All.

That night shines as one of the most profound realizations of my life. It shifted my spiritual practice completely — away from practicing like a man and toward trusting my own path. It proved to me that I could trust my SHE's guidance and the boons that my own feminine realization could have, in both my own life and the lives of others. Over the years since that night, I've been able to unpack its significance more and more, like the gradual decoding of a life-altering dream.

I now realize that what allowed so much to shift for me that week was releasing my black-and-white thinking. When I embraced paradox (going to stay with monks to find the Feminine Face of God), fresh insight could pour in. We all experience this flash of clear understanding through the archetype of the Dakini. Here's a story that illustrates her magic, the transformation I experienced at St. Benedict's, and the imminent initiation that awaits us next.

Machig Labdrön, an eleventh-century Tibetan yogini who was an expression of the Great Mother of Wisdom, underwent an initiation with her teacher. In the midst of receiving his teachings, she magically rose and spontaneously began to dance in midair. Next, she flew through the walls of the temple, high up into the branches of a tree that hovered over a pond near the monastery, remaining there in a state of deep meditation.

Lama Tsultrim, the modern-day emanation of Machig Labdrön, recounts,

> The pond was the residence of a powerful *naga*, or water
> spirit. These capricious, mythic beings are believed to

cause disruption and disease when disturbed, and can also act as treasure holders or protectors when they are propitiated.... [They are] so terrifying that the local people did not even dare to look at the pond, never mind approach it.[1]

The water spirits below considered Machig's arrival to be a direct confrontation, so they approached her menacingly. Unperturbed, she remained in meditation, which only made them more irate. When they teamed up to try to overwhelm her, Machig simply transformed her body into a food offering for the nagas. Their aggression immediately evaporated, and they aligned with Machig, vowing to forever protect and serve her.

Lama Tsultrim explains that by extending compassion to the demons and offering her body as food (rather than fighting with them), Machig transformed her demons into her allies.[2]

Like Machig, when we offer ourselves in love to the shadow dimensions of our own psyches that we've warred with for our entire lives, we at last meet our greatest allies, our daemons.

Chapter 9

Unveiling the Sacred Heart
of *Real* Feminine Power

Watch the ones whose only option left is to lean into the questions.
The ones who are uninhibited by the unknown because they've jumped
into that gaping hole and found themselves, by grace, unswallowable.
Watch the ones who willingly stand with feist and say, 'I feel it all,'
even when it scares the shit out of them. It's not brave to have answers.

— Mandy Steward, *Spiritual Wanderings*

I'll go ahead and say it since you're all thinking it anyway. Right about...
here...you want to call it quits. You get cold feet before your wedding, feel
like you'd rather stay home than go on the big trip you've been planning for
months, or, during the transition phase of labor, wonder if you could just
not do this whole baby thing after all. Your Inner Skeptic takes center stage,
grabs the bullhorn, and quips, *Haven't we come far enough? Do we* really *want*
this? Want to just turn around and pour us a nice, big glass of wine instead?

Doubt works in cahoots with our Skeptics. They rally the troops:
our Inner Critics and Patriarchs, perhaps our Perfectionists and Pushers.
Through slanderous self-talk, they mobilize our destructive habits, at-
tempting to divert our marches into the great unknown. When we creep

toward the crux of transformation and our bodies and psyches sense the nearness of a cataclysmic shift, they want us to run — *really* fast and *really* far — in the *opposite* direction.

Luckily we've been practicing relaxing into intensity and annihilation during our SHE Cycles. We've also learned that these inner selves are simply doing their jobs by protecting our tender cores, because what's more vulnerable than stepping off the cliff's edge into an eerie chasm of uncertainty?

Here's all you need to recognize to take the next step: It's *okay* to be afraid. It's *okay* to not know. It's *okay* to want to turn back. We *all* experience fear and doubt in the face of not knowing. The closer you are to the nexus of your transition, the stronger your fear and doubt will be, because that's also the point of your greatest potential for change. Pause and recognize this. Allow the immense discomfort to be there. Rather than running from or numbing to it, open to it. Quaking in your (sexy) boots is required. In so doing, you'll invite in grace — that magical ingredient that allows the phoenix to rise from the ashes, the butterfly to emerge from the chrysalis, and the baby to stretch its neck out from the birth canal.

You're ready. You've got this. Uncertainty isn't here to antagonize you; it's a good friend, here to *help* you. Without it, you would never try anything new. Would you have become a mother, gotten married, remodeled your house, started that business, even embarked on a spiritual path, if you had known beforehand what it would demand of you? Probably not! You *need* uncertainty, because it fuels you to try new things. It keeps you contributing to the greater good by continually taking risks throughout your life.

To conduct our initiation from fear and uncertainty to faith and power, let's call in the help of a mighty — and mostly unknown — feminine archetype: the Dakini.

Invoking the Dakini Principle

As Marion Woodman explains in *Dancing in the Flames*,

> [In] almost all stories of great saints in Tibet, the dakini appears at crucial moments. The encounters often have

a quality of sharp, incisive challenge to the fixated con-
ceptions of the practitioner. They may occur through a
human dakini, or through a dream or mirage-like appearance which vanishes after the message is communicated.
These encounters often have a grounding, practical in-
sightful quality that is sharp and wrathful. This is the
primordial raw energy of the dark goddess....By breaking through the either/or rigidities, the Black Goddess
creates the space for spontaneity, for new experience, for
new insight.[1]

Here's a story to help us see how the Dakini principle can appear unexpectedly in our daily lives.

A monk in ancient India entered into a solitary retreat. Since the
monk felt like he was on the cusp of a breakthrough, his teacher advised
him to do a *sadhana* for the Tantric female Buddha of wild wrath, Vajrayogini, during his retreat. One day, deep in meditation, he heard his door
open. Turning around, he saw a beautiful young maiden walk in from the
courtyard beyond his room.

"Women aren't supposed to be in here!" he shouted. Then he saw
that she carried with her a piece of bloody meat — something he knew he
couldn't eat because of his monastic vows.

Ignoring his protests, she walked closer to him. "I slaughtered this for
you," she insisted, extending the red carcass to him, a symbolic gesture
that was part of a larger offering to him: dining on meat, drinking wine,
and engaging in sexual union.

This only made the monk even more irate. "Please go immediately
and leave me to my retreat! You're not supposed to be here! Leave right
now!" he demanded in horror, completely forgetting that the very practices he was immersed in were in service of invoking this wild, enlightened
feminine.

She obeyed his wishes and left, and the monk completed his retreat.

Afterward, he visited with his teacher to debrief.

"Well, tell me, what happened on your retreat?" his teacher asked.

The monk answered, "Overall, it was really good. Nothing much happened. But, wait, actually, there was this *one thing* that happened with a young woman." And he went on to tell his teacher the whole story.

Afterward, his teacher stared at him sternly and growled, "Do you *know* who that was?!"

"No," the monk replied tepidly.

"Well, that was Vajrayogini herself, offering to initiate you into the depths of Tantric practice."

Shocked and taken aback, the monk immediately saw his mistake. He soon entered back into retreat, holding at the forefront of his awareness the intention to shift his rigid attitudes about good/bad and pure/impure that he held to so tightly. Eventually the woman appeared again, but this time as an old hag. Like the young maiden, she too offered him a feast.

This time he accepted, and his union with her brought him to complete realization.[2]

Such is the gift a Dakini can bring to dedicated practitioners on the brink of a breakthrough — but only when you invoke her and then have the eyes to see her.

I met my first Dakini in 2005 on the second floor of the Boulder Bookstore. Khandro Rinpoche, a respected Tibetan Buddhist teacher, was there giving a reading from her new book. Draped in her maroon robes, with her head shaved, she stood just below five feet tall. Still, her presence filled the entire room. Each of her words, punctuated with simple certainty and humble power, pierced me in the heart.

I want THAT, a voice bubbled up from deep within me.

Several years later, I trusted my intrigue in Khandro Rinpoche and went to stay for two weeks at her nunnery in the hills of Mussoorie, India. There I learned what her name, Khandro, really means. In Tibetan, the word for Dakini is *Khadro*, translated as a woman who moves through space, or a sky dancer. A Dakini is a female Buddha — the most important manifestation of the empowered, enlightened feminine in Tibetan Buddhism. Dakinis always appear in liminal, transitory moments: between life and death, sleeping and waking, day and night. You are most likely to see them in dreams at dawn or to see them at sunset. In fact, their secret, symbolic language of initiation is called "the twilight language."

Dakinis are first described in pre-Aryan goddess traditions as wild, wrathful carnivores who delivered important messages and teachings to great yogis in the places they practiced (and feared) most — cemeteries and charnel grounds. From this tradition, human Dakinis arose in ancient India. Highly realized female practitioners and spiritual teachers, they lived like nobility, for they were the only women who could own land.

They celebrated the sacredness of embodiment by transmuting erotic passion into sexual ecstasy and spiritual insight through intercourse with other male practitioners, serving as "sacred prostitutes," much like the courtesans of ancient Europe prior to the Inquisition. Around the eighth century, these Dakinis joined Buddhism, which was until then devoid of any female presence. From this mingling, Tantric Buddhism arose, spread up into Tibet, and became enfolded into the tradition of the Awakened feminine that we see today.

As modern female spiritual practitioners, we must call upon Dakinis during transitions and at the start of any creative project. Because they are gatekeepers at the threshold of great doubt, they guard the daemons of our innermost secret realms — genuine, embodied insight.

In true feminine fashion, they most enjoy mischievously delivering their wisdom through play and trickery. If the Dakini notices that we're getting too controlling, serious, and fixated on dualistic, overly rational, black-and-white thinking, she's the first one to shake things up. She pulls the rug out from underneath us, turns our worlds upside down, and forces us to relax our rigid preferences in order to *get the f'ing point.*

Like all the other inner selves we've visited, Dakinis aren't some exotic, external entity (although, like all other archetypes, they can and do appear externally). They're aspects of our own psyches that often serve as "midwives of the psyche...[guides] and [consorts] who [activate] intuitive understanding and profound awareness."[3]

Lama Tsultrim explains that, contrary to some of the West's most popular archetypes of the Sacred Feminine, which are serene and merciful like the Madonna, Dakinis express the ever-changing, wild, active, and free aspect of the feminine that animates emptiness — and is therefore an energy that every practitioner must also open to for realization. If we don't actively work with this wild dimension of feminine energy within our own psyches, it becomes subversive, transforming into more of the

Witch archetype. We must draw this energy out, using it to fuel an expression of feminine enlightenment that currently doesn't exist in the world that gravely needs it.

During times that you feel you've reached rock bottom in your transition, and you know that the only way to go is up, call on the Dakini within you. Remember that she likes to play and may appear in a form that challenges your worldview, as the young maiden did for the monk and the Golden Dakini at St. Benedict's monastery did for me.

Invite her in. She's here to gift you with your daemon. Are you ready for a taste of the empowered, enlightened feminine within you?

Listening in "the Between"

The Dakinis fly not only through the horizon at dusk, but also within the landscapes of our bodies. They beat their drums in our bellies and dance in the innermost chambers of our hearts. I once heard Dr. Christiane Northrup call these our "lower" and "upper" hearts, and Traditional Chinese Medicine termed the energetic superhighway between our hearts and wombs the Heart-Uterus, or Chong Mai, meridian.

Traveling through this inner, energetic pathway, the Dakinis force us to stop desexualizing our aliveness. Just as sexual intercourse is needed for conception, we need our untamed essence to fuel our transformations. In fact, all of our greatest life initiations transpire within this circuit between our yonis and our hearts: experiencing menarche, losing virginity, consummating marriage, giving birth, breastfeeding, and undergoing menopause. These sexual, embodied experiences are the most profoundly spiritual and transformative events of our lives. Feminine empowerment isn't a static, secular affair. It's profoundly spontaneous and erotic.

When we travel up this vertical access from our wombs and into our hearts, holding the intention that all of our actions flow from a sense of inner harmony, we're now able to see with the eye our hearts. As Cynthia Bourgeault teaches in her book *The Meaning of Mary Magdalene*, "The heart is not the seat of one's personal emotional life, but an organ of spiritual perception.... The heart is primarily an instrument of sight — or *in*sight."[4] There, like Jesus on the crucifix, we surrender our egos, understanding that love alone can finish this journey, for it's love that ultimately heals and persists beyond the death of our egos. This crucial shift in our perception transpires within what author Sera Beak calls "the between" and what ancient Gnostic traditions term the *nous* (pronounced "noose").[5]

Here's how Sera Beak defines the between:

> A dimension often forgotten.... In the ancient world, the *nous* was seen as "the finest point of the soul...." It gives us access to the intermediate realm between the purely sensory and the purely spiritual.... This is the space I've visited since I was a child to "be with" God.... This is my soul's space. In fact, it is *through* my soul that I enter this space.... What I Receive In this Space doesn't always make sense, but It always Makes Love. When I'm in this space, it's less like a psychic "seeing" and more like a heart knowing. I do not go up and out to receive the goods; I go down and in... [to] a blazing point *between* my head and my lower body, behind my heart, disclosing not my heart chakra but what I call the Heart of my heart.[6]

Platonic traditions define the nous as "the mind," whereas Gnosticism and eastern wisdom traditions view it as a property of "the heart." We can't force or will our way into the nous. Grace lets us in, arising out of prolonged, deep stillness through meditation, or in moments of poignant awe when our mental commentary and sense of self completely fall away.

Unfortunately, through prizing more scientific, rational views of the world over more subtle, intuitive ones, we've lost the faith, and therefore the capacity, to experience the nous through communing with our everyday lives. This is not unlike how the monk lost the ability to see the Dakini in the maiden.

We've all experienced this "between" space before, especially in our youth when we more freely engaged in the transcendental. My visions of Mother Mary as a child and my grown-up visitations from Mary Magdalene transpired in the nous. It's the very space we've been working on opening and trusting during our time in our SHE space. Emerging as flashes of premonition, visions, and instantaneous full-body insights, these mystical openings allow us to commune with the divine directly. Every woman is capable of experiencing this direct revelation.

To clarify this a bit further, let's add a dash of *neti neti*, a Sanskrit expression that means "not this, not this." Here are some things that the nous is *not*:

- A hallucination
- A visualization, daydream, or fantasy
- A dialogue with one of your inner selves
- A memory
- An emotional release
- A facsimile of a spiritual insight that you heard about from someone else
- A preexisting concept or expectation for how you "should" experience the divine

The mind cannot comprehend the nous — only the heart can *experience* it. In an era that overvalues certainty, welcome your confusion. It's the doorway to insight.

Up until now we've been working on strengthening the containers of our bodies and psyches so they will be able to *stay* in the nous. We can't force it; we can only create the conditions for it. As Cynthia Bourgeault explains,

> The inner precondition for all visionary communication is a capacity to remain emotionally rock-steady, not allowing any wave of psychic excitation to ruffle the still waters on which the image will reflect. Any "Oh wow! Is this really happening?"; any curiosity ("How is it happening?"); any craving or excitement — and the vision is gone.[7]

As we saw in my grace-filled yoga practice at the Snowmass monastery, we don't know when insight will strike or when our prayers will be answered. Continuing our practice, staying receptive, and keeping our hearts open is the best we can do. We put in our time, and grace does the rest.

Holding Steady at Your Honest Edge

As Pema Chödrön, the author of *When Things Fall Apart*, explains,

> In Tibetan there's an interesting word: *ye tang che*. The *ye* part means "totally, completely," and the rest of it means "exhausted." Altogether, *ye tang che* means totally tired out. We might say "totally fed up." It describes an experience of complete hopelessness, of completely giving up hope. This is an important point. This is the beginning of the beginning. Without giving up hope — that there's somewhere better to be, that there's someone better to be — we will never relax with where we are or who we are.[8]

From this place of no clear exit, a creative solution — one that is just right for you — *will* emerge. However, this will only occur if you stay present to the opposing energies that feel as though they are at war within you. You must step out of your comfort zone and from who you usually are in your day-to-day life. It's not easy, but in reinventing yourself, you will release astonishing amounts of healing, creative energy — the same energy that used to haunt you will soon sustain your new life.

To survive the inner war between heaven and hell, you must touch *everything* in this world with your heart, without closing. *This* is feminine realization. Being available to life's full range — from the most grotesque to the most beatific — is true feminine devotion. The more intimate you are with your edges — the precise peak levels of intensity that you can stand without harming yourself — the more alive you feel. There, you are free of who you have been, wondrous with not yet knowing who you are becoming.

Because we're so stuck in our old ways, we often need big jolts to wake us out of our trances. Skilled teachers and life crises can offer this, because they teach us that real practice begins when we collapse in an exhausted heap. Up until that point, we use skillful means to "do" things to help us change. Then, when we finally reach that place where we want to give up, it's time to enter our hearts and surrender to the practice of "not doing." With steady devotion to what and whom we cherish most, we let go and allow. It's time to give what we've been trying to open the chance to open us instead.

When this initiation occurs, the tremendous life force energy that has been locked inside the demonic impulse is freed. This period of dissolution, which looks different for everyone (as does the outcome), requires a strong inner container, and an attitude of acceptance, curiosity, and willingness. It demands that we let go of step-by-step formulas and instead follow the unpredictable creative impulse of life all the way to the resurrection in our hearts.

Riding the Edge of Your Transformation

Here are some steps to take when approaching the apex of your initiation.

1. Identify your edges. Know the difference between pain and intensity. The goal is to feel your maximum intensity without being in pain. List all the areas in your life where you feel that intensity through being challenged and tested. What's your edge in physical fitness? What yoga poses do you find most challenging? Where do you collapse in your relationships, health, work, finances, life purpose, and creativity? What emotions and mental states can you not tolerate? Rather than waging hidden battles with these edges, bring them to the forefront. Here, they're ripe for change.

2. Explore your relationship to your edge. Do you tend to push yourself past your edge, often finding yourself in crisis as a result? Or do you shy away from it, preferring not to "rock the boat"? When you *are* at your edge, how do you react? In a yoga pose, do you push past it and injure yourself? Do you say "that's not for me" and do something else? Do you burn out from overworking, or deaden yourself from your lack of effort?

3. When you're at your edge, engage your meditative awareness, rather than your usual modes of reactivity. Employ all the methods we've explored so far — from attunement, to mindfulness, to working with challenging emotions. Draw on all your inner resources here. If you want a different outcome at your edge, you need to use different methods. Fear is usually just a series of thoughts, so stay with the rawness of your sensation.

4. Cultivate a mood of compassion and gratitude. A miracle can arise when we engage our minds to reframe within an inner disposition of love whatever is occurring. Compassion triggers insight and opening. Embrace your entire experience with a mother's love. Feel gratitude for your challenges. What have they taught you? Who have they helped you to become? Anything that we can't accept about ourselves cannot be transformed.

5. Commune with your edge from your courageous heart. Now, *physically* activate your heart. Take a breath over the front surface of your heart, and love your limitations from your heart. Keep breathing from your heart into whatever you find challenging.

6. Stay. Don't run. Right when you're about to have a breakthrough, your ego puts up a huge fight or orders you to run. Whatever you do, just stay! Practice mind over matter. You are way stronger and more powerful than you could ever give yourself credit for. Imagine all of your teachers, mentors, allies, family members, friends, and top cheerleaders circled around you. When you don't think you can do it, imagine them rooting for you.

7. Tremble, and say YES. Shaking is a great sign. It means that blockages are clearing and healing energy is moving through your body in a new way. Trust that this is the grace of the Goddess flowing through you. *As long as it's arising from intensity, not pain, this energy won't hurt you.* Trust it, and keep opening to it. This is new life flowing in. This is your daemon. Say YES!

8. Flame the fire of your devotion. Before we can step over the threshold of our edge into our new life, we have to sacrifice some aspect of our previous one. No false expressions of power can be maintained as you cross over. Relieve yourself of anything that you are unwilling to tolerate and no longer need. Then give everything in your felt awareness away, from your heart, as a gift — who you've been, your expectations about who you will become, your challenges and blessings. Remember the bigger picture about why you're on this journey. Call upon your devotion. What are you dedicated to that's greater than you? See that meeting your edge is a gesture of love, rather than a militant attempt at perfection.

9. Trust and surrender. It takes tremendous strength and integrity to surrender, rather than buying into our fears. Keep traveling on the high road. Don't turn away. For whatever you release, you're always given something back ten-thousand-fold.

10. Allow grace to open you. The key word here is *allow* — not *try* or *force*. Ultimately, we can't open ourselves. Get clear on your edge, stay lovingly with it past the point of what feels comfortable, and through that, allow your challenges to be taken away from you. Trust in divine timing to bring your salvation at the perfect moment, in the perfect way. Open yourself to this possibility and be surprised and amazed at how it unfolds, for this deep purification transpires differently for each of us. We often think that change requires so much effort, but this requires no effort at all. Take your seat in the deepest part of you, activate the wisdom of your heart, and allow your own true nature that's always running toward you to blossom from within.

To practice these steps, choose a yoga posture to hold for three minutes. I recommend a squat pose, which is also what I'll use here as an example. Before coming into it, set a timer for three minutes.

To come into the squat pose, first stand up and place your feet hip-distance apart, with the outer edges of your feet parallel. Bend your knees until your thighs are parallel to the floor. Lift your arms in front of you, elbows softly bent and middle fingers pointing toward each other like you're hugging an invisible tree.

Breathe with your mouth closed, the tip of your tongue resting behind your upper row of teeth. Stay in the pose for the full three minutes. If you absolutely have to come out of it, do so slowly and calmly, without reactivity. As you ride the waves of intensity, conduct your energy and awareness, following the previous steps internally.[9]

Unveiling Your Sacred Heart

So far on our journey we've worked with the two main energy centers in the body that I mentioned in chapter 2: the belly and the solar plexus. Now, when we open at our edges, we at last inhabit the space where our initiation will transpire — our hearts.

Last summer I traveled to Chicago to visit my mom and sisters and to shop for a wedding dress together. Despite the cliché this rite of passage has become, nothing could have prepared me for the elation of dressing as a bride for the first time. My youngest sister, Anne, who had gotten married the year before, advised that I try on *all* the different silhouettes: ball gown, A-line, trumpet, mermaid, and sheath.

"You'll be surprised what you end up liking! Usually it's not what you think," she urged.

During one of my countless struts along the invisible runway from my dressing room to the fitting pedestal, where my ooh-ing and ah-ing entourage awaited, Anne walked toward me with a veil.

"Just give it a whirl," she smiled with a wink, plunking it down on my crown.

"No. No way. Uh-uh," I protested. I had never, *ever* wanted a veil. I thought they seemed so stodgy and old-fashioned. But, as I turned around to look at my reflection in the mirror, I gasped. Then I smiled and jumped up and down in unbridled glee. My mother and sisters joined me in this unexpected celebration.

"See, Sara!" Anne laughed. "That's how I felt at my wedding! It's like I *became a bride* when I put on a veil. There's just something to it. Weird, right?"

That day I discovered that veils really *do* hold a uniquely feminine mystique. They guard the delicate boundary between the seen and unseen.

There's an adage in Sufi Islam that says that the soul is covered by one thousand veils. Our lives, then, consist of endless unveilings. Every obstacle we face along our journeys offers us the chance to remove one of those veils. Our initiations are revelations, a word that derives from *revelare*, meaning "to draw back the veil," and they transpire in the heart, which has long been seen as the place of divine integration between spirit and matter, heaven and earth.

In Sanskrit, the word for the heart center, *anahata*, translates as "unstuck," for it's the place within us that's forever untouched by any wounding. Chinese and Ancient Egyptian religions believed the soul resided in the heart, yet these ancient teachings profoundly contradict the views of the modern world. In fact, one of the dangers of living estranged from feminine wisdom is that we've forgotten how to revere our own sacred hearts. Today, one in three women dies from heart disease, making it the number one killer for women.[10]

Even though we've largely forgotten its metaphysical magnificence, the heart continues to work ceaselessly for us, beating up to 40,000 times a day, 14.6 million times a year. Long identified as the center of the body, the heart is the first organ to develop in utero. Even though the heart only grows to be the size of a fist, it still transmits the most powerful electromagnetic field in the body, with an amplitude sixty times greater than that of the brain!

About 65 percent of the heart is composed of neurons.[11] It contains its own form of intelligence and serves as both the key to our human bonding and the medium through which we commune with the cosmos. This electromagnetic field lives in the realm of subtle energy and serves as a matrix, housing our cosmic interconnectedness and providing a life-sustaining net for all that is. It allows everything to evolve and thrive, and to decay and pass away. Like a gigantic spider web, there's no end or beginning to this matrix. Wherever you are in it, it is both your entry point and the center of the universe.

When we fully inhabit our place in this universal matrix, and our egos surrender to our SHEs, we land in the dominion of true feminine power: eternal, Absolute love. From here, we discover a tremendous love for life, just as it is. There's no good or bad, right or wrong. Only love streams out in all directions — saturating every part of us fully. Even though our deepest wounds may never fully heal, activating our hearts awakens miracles, allowing lifelong obstructions to dissolve instantaneously. Unshackled by past burdens, we know, without a doubt, that no matter what transpires, we're always, ultimately, okay.

A few years ago, while teaching a weekend retreat at the Shambhala Mountain Center here in Colorado, I experienced one such magical heart revelation. For a few days I felt sharp pains in my heart, something that wasn't unusual for me at that time. This transpired during the phase I wrote about in the Introduction, when I often had intense, energetic, Kundalini experiences (the awakening of the Goddess within as energy that moves like a snake from the base of the spine to the crown of the head, often as a result of deep, spiritual practice). As we've explored, I had previously experienced this energy when it moved through my belly as rage while I worked with my therapist Diana, then through my solar plexus as repressed power. Now it was piercing my heart.

There wasn't much I could do about these experiences except allow the energy to release and move. However, by the end of the retreat the pain in my heart wasn't subsiding, so, after I went home, I visited my acupuncturist for help.

"Did anything unusual happen while you were teaching?" he asked, moving around the table, lifting one wrist and then the other, closing his eyes and listening to my pulse.

"What do you mean?"

"Sometimes when you're serving others and you start to move more energy through you, you can put more strain on your heart. Did you experience anything like that during your retreat?"

I scrunched up my forehead. "Um, no." I felt confused. "Nothing different from how any of my other retreats are. Nothing out of the ordinary."

"Are you sure?" he probed.

I started to feel annoyed. *Why is he asking me all these questions about the weekend?* I thought to myself. *What does that have to do with anything?*

But I ultimately trusted his inquiry and started to think back through each day, through each hour of each day, to see if I was forgetting anything. *Ohhh...* I thought, suddenly remembering a moment that perhaps I had written off too lightly.

"Well," I shared, "I *did* take a walk, by myself, up to the stupa on Saturday evening. I circumambulated it, making the declaration that I'm ready to make a greater contribution, and that I need more support in order to do that. I prayed, *Whatever arises, may it awaken my heart, and may this life be of benefit to all beings.*"

"That's it," my acupuncturist confirmed. "That's what I thought. I'm not getting that anything's physically wrong here, or that your heart is in any danger. It feels like more energy is trying to come through and it's getting all jammed up in your chest and your left shoulder. So I'll put some needles in, and we'll try to free up this energy and smooth it out. Sound good?"

I nodded, closing my eyes and remembering conversations I'd had with Sofia during other times of transition. She often instructed: "If this is happening, it must be good."

He then left me alone, with the needles in, to drift off to sleep. Several minutes later, I woke up to a serene warmth in my heart. The pain had completely dissipated. With my eyes closed, I felt the shores of the two hemispheres of my body parting, my heart widening. Between them, a pink river of ecstasy flowed down into my belly, through the mouth of my yoni, between my feet, communing with the early spring branches beyond them.

The ecstasy and love were too great to hold back. *This feels so good!* I giggled to myself as I rocked my head from side to side in sublime pleasure. Streams of rainbow-colored light spread out from my heart and filled the room.

My acupuncturist came back in fifteen minutes later. "How are you doing in here?" he asked.

"*Really* good," I replied, eyes still closed, grinning widely.

"I thought that might be the case." He added, "I'll leave you here a bit longer, then."

My whole body became a heart. From within, SHE boomed, "This, right here, is feminine power. *Feminine power is LOVE.*"

Your Ritual to Leave the Underworld

Reading about this initiation isn't enough; you have to experience it for yourself. Remember: there can never be a rebirth without a death. To depart from the underworld, you must purify your heart and let go. Take your time with this.

- Whom do you need to forgive?
- What messes do you need to clean up?

- What roles, identities, beliefs, and activities do you need to let go of?
- What lessons did you learn here in the underworld?
- Find gratitude for what you already have. Create a list of your blessings and let a feeling of thankfulness permeate your entire body.
- Select something that feels precious to you and ceremoniously give it to someone who would love and need it, or leave it somewhere in nature. Both methods symbolize your offering to your SHE.

Receive Permission from the Dark Goddess to Ascend

To listen to this visualization, go to www.TheBookofSHE.com/practices to download the audio file. I've also included it in written form here. Make sure you have your journal and a pen or pencil nearby before you begin.

Come into a comfortable seat. Close your eyes. Take five slow, deep, and even breaths, inhaling for a count of five and exhaling for a count of five. Let your mind follow each breath. Inhale into any physical tension you feel. Exhale, release it. Inhale into any preoccupying emotions. Exhale, release them. Inhale into any thoughts or dominant mind forms. Exhale, release them. Inhale into any sounds or distractions in the room. Exhale, release them. Inhale into your whole body. Exhale, release.

Next, get in touch with your earthing cord (from chapter 2). Feel a thick cord extending from your belly down into the center of the earth. Clearly envision each end of the cord. Inhale earth energy up through your feet and legs, as well as through this cord. Exhale and store it in your belly. Breathe in that way a few more times. Then widen and strengthen your earthing cord until you feel a steady flow of surplus earth energy flowing through your body. If at any time you start to feel distracted or overwhelmed during this visualization, reestablish your grounding.

Now imagine your inner home and see yourself back in the cellar. Bring this dark dungeon back into all of your senses. What does it smell like? What's the temperature? What do you see around you? You can always pause here if you need more time to envision it.

Now, look again to the darkest corner of the cellar. Down on the floor, revisit the worse version of yourself possible — who you would be if everything had gone wrong in your life and your demons possessed you. Get a clear picture of your own dark sister here.

When she comes fully into view, see her physical form dissolving into a mirage of black smoke. From that, see her becoming the Dark Goddess herself. Give yourself some time here, until the Dark Goddess, as she appears to you, comes fully into view.

When you're ready, slowly walk toward the Dark Goddess. Ask her if she has anything she needs to tell you before you leave her domain. Pause and listen. She might speak in words, sounds, movement, symbols, or just a feeling you get from being with her. Again, if you need more time, pause until you feel complete with this step.

Receive what she has to say, and also take some time to ask her any other questions you have for her. When you feel complete, thank her for the lessons of the underworld. Look down in your hands and see a gift that you have, an offering for her. Trust whatever you see and extend it toward her.

Then ask for her permission to return to the light. When and if she grants it, step into her, acknowledging that she is part of you. She is your dark side, your dark sister. Welcome any fear or intensity that arises. Fully intermingle with and dissolve into the Dark Goddess. Feel and see whatever happens next.

If she doesn't grant your permission, ask what else needs to transpire for you to leave the underworld.

If she does, as soon as this merging feels complete, look around the underworld of your inner cellar and say goodbye. Slowly walk back up the stairs, leaving the door open behind you. Return to the ground floor of your home. Feel the light of day hitting your skin, both in your inner home, and in the room around you right now.

When you feel ready, take some deeper breaths and slowly open your eyes.

Write down what transpired during your time with the Dark Goddess and leaving the underworld. Write for at least ten minutes without stopping. Keep your pen moving with the stream of your consciousness, describing everything you can remember about your time down in your cellar.

Take one last look around. Praise the darkness for allowing you to commune with your own sacred heart. When you feel complete, it's time to ascend.

Journaling Questions

- In retrospect, where have you seen the Dakini principle in action in your life?
- How do you react — physically, emotionally, and mentally — when you're at your edge?
- When in your life have you fully surrendered, and what was that like? If you've never experienced that, what scares you about surrender?
- What would it look like for you to feel your current challenges from your heart, rather than analyzing them with binary thinking?

Part IV

The Ascent

*I have a feeling that my boat
has struck, down there in the depths,
against a great thing.*
*And nothing
happens! Nothing...Silence...Waves...*

*— Nothing happens? Or has everything happened,
and are we standing now, quietly, in the new life?*

—Juan Ramón Jiménez, "Oceans," translated by Robert Bly

The Temple Priestess

These next steps on our journey might shock — or even anger — you. If this happens, go at your own pace in a way that feels right. I encourage you to remember that our gold lies in the dark. If we succumb to conventional, binary thinking and deny the darkness, we split ourselves off from our power and potential.

It would be wonderful if we could always be nice girls who take lavender baths when we get really upset, or channel our energy into yoga, journaling, and creative expression — all things I advocate. When we can practice these healthy and self-affirming activities, that's wonderful. But the feminine isn't all light and joy, sweetness and mothering.

We've seen how Dakinis and sacred prostitutes, which have also been called Temple Priestesses, expressed and shared their enlightenment through their bodies (whereas their male counterparts, or consorts, transmitted their wisdom through the fullness of their presence and awareness). These traditions teach that through her sexuality, a woman fully grounds into her divinity. Now it's time for us to learn how to do this too.

Today as modern women on spiritual paths, this aspect of our fruition is often omitted. It's lost, forgotten, and seldom spoken of. We instead follow a man's path — that of unmovable, pervasive (and in its unhealthy form, disembodied) awareness. We fail to see the topic of sexuality all the way back to its source — the blossoming of our hearts and bodies into the expression of our true nature of, and as, love.

It's time for us to start turning over the stones of our spirituality and sexuality simultaneously. In service of our evolution, this disowned aspect of our womanhood needs to be spoken of. We must earnestly and whole-heartedly practice with our hearts and yonis just as much as we do with our minds.

Today's Temple Priestess lives in the cellar of our collective uncon-scious but is emerging once again, although slowly. It's she who shares her body as an illuminating, enlivening offering for the benefit of all beings.

As a longtime feminist, I had always been repulsed by strip clubs and the abuse and exploitation I perceived women suffered there. However, as part of my own sexual exploration and reclamation of the Temple Priest-ess archetype, I felt I could finally hold the complexity of the adult danc-er's world without collapsing into judgment or despair.

I fully acknowledge that much darkness festers in strip clubs; yet, as with all things we're exploring, it's not a black-and-white topic. I'm here to point out a misunderstood side to this real-life underworld. There we can also find modern-day Temple Priestesses hiding out, bringing light into the dark, through their sacred and sexual bodies.

Recently, I have taken some of my most advanced students to ex-perience this revelation for themselves. However, it was during my first visit to a strip club that I initially received my healing transmission from a Temple Priestess who was embodied as a sly, sensual, and heavily tattooed brunette. She held the salve that I, and so many of us, desperately need.

As we proceed, please notice and own your judgments. Take 100 per-cent of the responsibility for your experiences. Stay open and curious. My story, which follows, points to the need for us, as women, to create sacred spaces where, once again, the Temple Priestess can love and dance — beyond strip clubs, prostitution, Burning Man, or pole-dancing classes. She is ready to emerge in full daylight, not as an object but as a liberator, goddess, and healer.

As women we can't always just look to our partners to unchain our sexuality. We also must look to other women, and to expressing this part of ourselves in the safe company of our soul sisters.

Now I offer to you my story, as an inspiration and provocation for inviting her medicine back into your life too.

Boulder, Colorado; September 4, 2013

"I want to go to the strip club," I blurted out.

"Are you *sure*?" Keith asked, excited but circumspect. "You have to be prepared for a lot of dark energy. You sure you're up for it?"

I looked away and paused. Then looked back and declared, "Yes, I am ready for it." And I was.

Holding hands, we sauntered down Pearl Street, around a corner, across an alley. We flashed IDs to a bouncer and then made our way down a dark flight of stairs. A young Asian man stood behind the counter. Signs around him shouted the rules: "No photography. No videos." I felt a tinge of jealousy that Keith had been there before — that he was comfortable in the dark with his sexuality, like this. Then we walked inside the club, and it wasn't at all what I expected. The movies always show a stage, a catwalk, bright lights, leggy showgirls, leering men. This was just a ring for ordinary women to writhe around in plastic stilettos.

"It's best to sit back here." Keith guided us, rolling two armchairs atop the red carpet until they sat side by side.

I crossed and then uncrossed my legs, planting my black high heels firmly on the floor, knowing full well how awkward and uptight I looked. *Relax*, I kept telling myself. *Shift your hips. Move a little. Don't freeze up.* I wondered if anyone I knew would see me there.

"There, some seats have opened up. Let's get closer," Keith urged, grabbing my hand.

We sat at the edge of the stage, ringed by men as well as a surprising number of women. Two poles poked through the center, one at either end. Every several minutes, two new women appeared, first peeling off thin layers of clothing and then tauntingly taking their positions. Their hands gripped and legs wrapped around poles, seemingly lost in a state of rapture — even though I could tell they really weren't. Most seemed to be hiding inside a shell, caught in the two-dimensional illusion of their own objectification. They were gone — dreaming of somewhere else — their faces carefully constructed, sexualized masks, hiding whatever storm was raging beneath. My heart ached. Yet I also envied them, for a secret part of me longed to be on that stage too. To become the Goddess, not the object.

Keith put a few one-dollar bills down on the counter in front of me. "When you see a woman you like, you put this down in front of you, and she'll come over."

A song or two later, a different creature than the others came out. She had cropped dark-brown hair, curled at the ends. Tattoos across pale skin. A rose on her back. A shield on her right arm, a vine on her left. She wore a red knit tank-top dress that fell just below her derrière. She stopped and wiggled out of her dress, stripping down to just a G-string. Hips jiving right and left, she made her way toward me, thumbs hooked inside the strings of her panties. Teasingly, she pulled them part way down. Then she stood in front of me. Keith continued to watch but had moved carefully and quietly away, forgotten.

Her eyes were alive, and her smile reached out of her heart with a playful invitation. Uninhibited, bold, brave, and sexy. Very, *very* sexy. She crawled over the counter, and all the way onto my lap. Knees straddling my thighs, she was truly enjoying herself. Yes, she knew how powerful she was!

"What's your name?" I whispered. The goddess's lips curled in a smile. She placed her mouth on my ear and answered, "Dahlia."

"Can I touch you?" I asked.

Dahlia nodded.

I combed a hand through Dahlia's hair, tousling it and pulling it back at the hairline with some force. I then slid my hands around her back, along her waist, and between her soft inner thighs. We tapped into a shared current of erotic play where two bodies become one, dancing in turn on, one steady stream of feminine power unleashed. I had crossed the threshold, no longer stiff and stuck up, and now all I could do was flow, breathe, feel, and receive. *So this is what it's like to love a woman. God, this feels so good.*

"You're so gorgeous," Dahlia whispered to me. "And you smell so good. Thank you."

Pulling away, Dahlia gathered up the bills and strapped them inside her panties. She flitted away, on to the next pile of money, swallowed by the dark at the opposite end of the stage.

Keith leaned back into view. Keith! I had forgotten about him.

"You two really had a connection! Do you want to try a VIP dance with her? Just the two of you. No one watching. If you want one, I can call her back over," he offered.

"Yes, I want one," I answered, all body, no thought.

He somehow got Dahlia's attention as she slipped by several minutes later. "Two dances, for my lady here?" he asked.

"Oh," Dahlia said, "for her?" That smile came to her lips again. "I would be happy to."

Dahlia led me into the unlit back corner of the club, to an oversized velour loveseat whose back was high for privacy. I sat down, perched at the edge the seat, used to having a woman sit down next to me.

"No. Sit in the middle," Dahlia commanded. "Here. Like this." She took my hips and slid them to center.

A new song began, fast and electronic. Without missing a beat, Dahlia straddled me. I followed her lead. Hands over breasts, around belly, inner thighs, down the backs of legs. She bit my ear and nibbled my neck. I nuzzled my nose into her breasts. No giver, no receiver, but two women alive and in love. Not with each other, but with the erotic movement, in us, as us, between us, of life herself. We danced in and as the deep knowing of what being a woman is *really* about, I thought to myself, *My god, is this woman good. My god, am I good.*

When the song finally ended, Dahlia sat cradled, sideways on my lap, our arms wrapped around each other. The breath of two strangers, who were somehow now two lovers, intermingled in the air between us.

"That was amaaaazing," Dahlia whispered in my ear. "*You* are amazing."

"Thank you. Thank you so much. You're so beautiful," I responded.

"What's your name?" Dahlia asked.

"Sara," I revealed, feeling more of "me" coming back.

Dahlia stood up and reached her hand out to me to pull me up. Once on my feet, I tugged my shirt down and combed my fingers through my hair. Dahlia walked ahead of me, taking great, slinking strides in her stilettos. I moved behind her, emulating her poise and unflinching shine — not quite getting it, but much more than before. More than sex appeal, more than sexual energy, she had true *shakti*, and men and women both stepped respectfully out of her way as she moved through the crowd.

I returned to Keith, now sitting back from the stage, looking out from the shadows.

"How was it?"

"Awesome," I answered, still breathless. "Totally hot."

"Time to go, then?"

"Yes. Do you want a dance too?"

He shook his head.

Hand in hand we tucked out into the sharp night air. I smiled, smelling of Dahlia, the angel in the underworld who reminded me of my light.

Chapter 10

Turning On Your Brights

We never know how high we are / Till we are called to rise; /
And then, if we are true to plan, / our statures touch the skies

— *Emily Dickinson*

One drizzly Sunday morning, Arthur Miller parked in front of a pharmacy and opened the passenger-side door of his car. Out stepped his wife, Marilyn Monroe, although on that particular morning, she didn't look anything like Marilyn Monroe. Sick with a head cold, she looked like an average housewife, tired and washed out. She hid inside her oversized beige trench coat, covering her signature blonde locks with a white scarf.

Ten minutes later, filled prescription in hand, the pair headed back to their car. "MARILYN!" someone shrieked from across the street. "Hey! That's Marilyn Monroe!"

Passersby whizzed their heads around and darted toward the couple. In an instant, Marilyn switched her charisma on, sloughing her malaise and illuminating from within. She flashed her seductive smile. Her eyes sparkled. She posed for the cameras while flirting with her fans. That morning, Marilyn demonstrated her mastery of generously beaming her feminine radiance on the world. She went from hardly taking up *any* space to taking up every inch of it — and then some. In a nanosecond, she turned on her "brights" and *became* Marilyn.

Sofia shared this story with me a few years ago when I was learning how to "turn on my brights" and flip my own feminine radiance switch at will. Like most of us, I grew into womanhood harboring a deep confusion about my beauty and sexuality. Sometimes I needed to cloak it to keep me safe on New York City streets late at night, sometimes I used it to manipulate others to feel better about myself, and sometimes I pushed it away and shut it down because I didn't know how to absorb all the attention coming my way. I was a victim to my radiance, rather than the masterful conductor of it.

Marilyn represents an archetype of embodied, feminine love-light that we can *all* learn from and call upon. As Patriarchy's Daughters, we initially learned to fuel ourselves through our willpower and personas alone. But Marilyn reminds us that the art and science of joyfully partaking in life through beaming our great feminine strengths of love, ecstasy, and beauty, *in the presence of others*, is our sacred responsibility.

Be the Lover

I'm the first to admit that women who are drawn to feminine spiritual practice usually bring a deeply ingrained seriousness. It takes *a lot* of steadfastness to stay this course — not just for a week or month, but for our *entire* lives. And perhaps we've perpetuated that somberness by spending too much time in zendos or ashrams. We've ended up believing that the more austere we are, the more spiritually evolved we must be.

Feminine spiritual practice, on the other hand, brings us more fully *into* life — not above it. It teaches us that the more we embrace our dark emotions, the more fully we can commune with pleasure. Here, celebration, delight, ecstasy, and fun are not deterrents or distractions on the path; they are portals — and necessities — into deeper insight and aliveness.

Since we're all born hardwired with a negativity bias, this can be challenging. Everywhere we look seems lacking. During even our peak life experiences, we remain distracted, feeling that somehow things *still* aren't quite right.[1] Given these facts about our neurology, we need to practice looking on the bright side in any moment by turning the majority of our attention (60 percent or more) toward what feels good and right. We need to stay awake to where we're pointing our energy and attention and, if needed, reroute it in more life-affirming directions — as Marilyn did, head cold and all.

Of course, this doesn't mean that we chase only bliss and harmony, as has become the preferred route in popular "supermarket spirituality." Instead, we make ourselves available to feel and participate in *everything* arising in the present moment, while magnifying what feels good throughout.

And let's be honest here. The energy that Marilyn — and the Dakini — emits is highly *sexual*. Electric and seductive, the very creative life-force energy that we woke up in the underworld is synonymous with our sexual energy. When unfrozen and brought into consciousness, this fuels our self-healing and our ability to wield our unique flavors of power in the world.

This can be hard to grasp at first, because as modern women, we put sexual energy into a neat little shoebox in the bedroom closet. We think, "Okay, sexual energy is a thing that happens when I'm wearing Victoria's Secret lingerie or on date night," when in fact it's infinitely *more* than that. Our sexual energy *is* life itself. We cannot draw boundaries between our Dark Goddess energy, sexual energy, creative energy, health and vitality, and spiritual energy — they are all one and the same. During our ascent, we need to recognize our innocent, luminous, erotic nature — not just with our minds, but also through our direct participation in life. Once our raw vitality wakes up from old trauma and frozenness, it melts into the nectar that transforms the darkness into light, spirit into matter.

When we were young, we quickly learned to mask our incandescence because it was unsafe or simply too much for others to stand — as it was for Cinderella's stepsisters. Just as we learned to slowly adjust our eyes to the dark, we also need to learn to slowly adjust our eyes to the *light*. Little by little, we'll practice getting more comfortable with truly being seen. Bit by bit, we'll open ourselves to receive regard from the world and to fully inhabit this dazzlingly embodied feminine power that resides within all of us. It's one thing to recognize our daemons, and it's another thing to actively extend them as a gift for the world. Our sexual energy is what will fuel this offering, ushering us successfully through our descents and onward toward our homecomings.

Great female mystics throughout time have paved the way for us in their teachings, revealing tales of taking on the divine as their "lovers." Lala, a fourteenth-century North Indian mystic, left an unhappy marriage to wander Kashmir, singing her praise for God as she went. In the 1600s, Spanish Carmelite nun St. Teresa of Avila wrote of her rapturous visions of Jesus. Mother Teresa demonstrated fierce, feminine love and communed with her Lord every time she solaced the untouchables in the slums of Calcutta. Sera Beak writes about her modern-day voyages into the archetype of the Sacred Prostitute in her spiritual memoir, *Red Hot and Holy*.

As women, do we not all harbor the capacity for such exultant unions with our beloveds? Deep down, don't we all really, really *want* this? We can get so attached to what's wrong with our lives that we completely miss what every religion and science in the world points back to: there is nothing *but* light. Use your own life to express this truth. Don't miss out on this precious opportunity to fully inhabit your own golden, radiant core.

This isn't about objectification or submission to another person's sexual agenda. While many of us do need to remember how to flip this switch internally, ultimately, radiance is an intrinsic part of our feminine nature. It arises naturally when you feel a deep sense of inner peace and self-love. Our time in the underworld teaches us what true self-esteem is, and once we taste this, we can no longer bear betraying and defiling our own innate greatness. The more we let go, the more radiant we will be. We've learned invaluable life lessons, made friends with our inner selves, and cherished the intelligence of our female bodies. We exude wisdom and now, during our ascents, joyfully move toward sharing this with the world — not because we want to be loved and approved of, but because it's the natural fruit of our inner work. Above all else, we must "be the lover." In order to heal the world, we must cherish it, sing to it, and celebrate it. Once we've tasted the depths of our own self-love, we can't help but become lovers to the world, loving *everything* and *everyone*, without exception, until it aches.

The Discipline of Ecstasy

Sweet Sara. That's what people always used to call me. It didn't matter where I went in the world — whether it was to visit a cousin in the Midwest, have tea with a girlfriend in Bangkok, or read a piece of fan mail from someone I'd never met before. Everyone I knew at some point arrived at "Sweet Sara" as my nickname. Don't get me wrong. I was flattered that others thought I was nice, thoughtful, present, and *sweet*. But I was tired of always being just *sweet*. Because *sweet* can also mean playing it safe. It meant I didn't ruffle anyone else's feathers. *Sweet* sometimes stopped me from taking a big risk publicly, falling flat on my face, and looking like a fool. *Sweet* could also mean feeling inhibited — from trying to fit into other people's agendas or from dimming my passion (or beauty, ambition, sensitivity, sexuality, whatever) so I didn't exclude or make someone feel uncomfortable.

And on top of that, I'm so much more than just *sweet*. And so are you. Let's explore the "so much more" that longs to be expressed and seen in all of us. This "so much more" is the sexy, sharp-toothed, fierce, and growling go-after-what-you-want ecstatic, erotic, lit up, and — most of all — turned-on parts of ourselves. It's all the edgy, uncomfortable, and vibrantly alive "what's next" parts of us that keep us passionate about our lives. It's treading a new frontier in womanhood, where we live our eroticism in an open and everyday way — on our yoga mats, in our relationships, walking down the street, cooking dinner, putting the kids to bed, or in a business meeting.

Rather than incessantly thinking there's something wrong with you, it's time to risk celebrating your greatness. Simply by being born a woman, you're luminous, delicious, and brilliant — beyond your ego, soul, SHE, or anything you've tried to acquire or cultivate. You can't "put on" your radiant nature or buy it in an expensive face cream. You can only acknowledge and participate in it, for it lives inside you, as real and tangible as your lungs or thighbones. Like anything else in life, your radiance only grows the more you remember and nurture it.

Along with Marilyn, Venus, who is the Roman goddess of grace and love (and an expression of the Greek goddess Aphrodite), serves as a powerful archetype for our emergence. Ascending from the frothy sea of primordial creation, Venus is born, poised on her half shell, graciously bearing spring blossoms and erotic innocence. This goddess of beauty and desire personifies both relative and Absolute love. The planet Venus is named after her, and the Sumerian goddess Inanna, who famously made her own journey into the underworld, is also closely related to the star Venus. Both appear to descend into the west and rise again in the east, linking the underworld with the heavens. Venus, then, is the bridge, guiding women to fluidly navigate the temporal seas of living our dreams.

Since we are composed of salt water that's surrounded by skin, we too could consider ourselves to be sea creatures. Like dolphins playing in the shimmers of ocean and sunlight, when we get more and more comfortable with our own embodiment, we discover a divine, ecstatic pulsation deep in our cores. This is the place where the waves of agony and ecstasy crest and crash within the singular ocean of bliss. At the depths of our true nature, pain and pleasure are one and the same. Here we discover a deeper dimension of self-soothing — the complete allowance of everything to be as it is, right here, in the natural, pulsating perfection of our own bodies. It's ecstatic to love the fear all the way out of our bodies, nurturing our traumas and wounds to the point of pleasurable fullness.

Commit to an Ongoing Ecstasy Practice

Since nature abhors a vacuum, it's time to include new, *better* activities and beliefs that affirm your innate splendor to take the place of what you let go of in the underworld. Dressing in beautiful clothes, enjoying great sex, dancing provocatively, hugging and kissing and teasing and flirting — these are all important gateways to our freedom. Yes, we need to know how to sit alone in still silence, being with ourselves just as we are. But we also need to stretch ourselves and extend some of the feminine gifts that our self-serving bad moods and low self-esteem often squash.

Goddesses are always depicted with lavish clothes, glistening jewels, and lustrous hair. It's good medicine for us to internalize the Goddess through the practice of sacred adornment. It uplifts us and others to dress to the nines, be generous with our radiance, and light up a room (or someone's day) with our smile. We've seen this in goddesses incarnate like Kate Middleton, Princess Diana, Michelle Obama, and Jackie Kennedy Onassis. Amid all of the world's darkness, it is our responsibility to nourish all beings through our unconditional, ceremonious disposition of magnanimous beauty.

What's a simple, accessible ecstasy practice that you can take on for the next month to give this a whirl? Daily ecstasy practices must be realistic and doable, while also bringing you to your appropriate edge. If you aim too high *or* too low, you'll set yourself up for failure. Remember: Practices are something that we do *whether or not* we feel like it. We show up for them, day after day, even when it's hard or we're crazy busy. Unlike meditation or attunement, where we sit with ourselves just as we are, with these particular practices, we need to move beyond our resistance to adopt the mindset of "Fake it till you make it." It doesn't matter how you feel about it; just do it.

I asked women in our SHE School to share what practices they tried. Here's what some of them had to say:

- Sleeping naked every night.
- Maintaining bold, flirty eye contact with strangers (men and women) if I feel they are checking me out.
- Waking early for self-pleasuring that lasts at least ten minutes a few times a week. (Morning sex is the best, even with myself!)
- Eating a piece of fresh fruit each day and being completely present while doing so, to fully experience the sensual nature of it.
- Standing naked in front of a full-length mirror to check myself out.
- Standing under a cold-water blast for one minute at the end of my morning shower.
- Massaging my breasts with coconut oil.
- Dancing, without stopping, for at least three minutes during my lunch break.
- Wearing sexy underwear. Or, even better, no underwear!
- Giving my man a blow job at least once a week.
- Styling my hair rather than tying it up in a ponytail every day.

- Throwing out my old nursing bras and wearing my more vampy, sexy heels on nights out.
- Wearing less spandex and yoga clothes and bringing a little more sass to my wardrobe to help my inner goddess feel adorned instead of so frumpy.
- Staying away from social media, which ultimately makes me feel empty. Instead, I'm going to take myself on more dates (solo)!

Going Deeper into Ecstasy

- Inquire into your Inner Seductress and the dominant Good Girl using the guidelines for working with your inner selves from chapter 6. Dialogue with this duo for a month, bringing the disowned self more into the light, while letting the more dominant self relax on the sidelines.
- Create a Pinterest board or paper collage for your Inner Seductress. Give her a name. Find role models — in the media, stories, and your life — for empowered, sex-positive women. My Inner Seductress is named Vixen, and you can see her on her Pinterest board (www.Pinterest.com/saraavantstover).
- Cut out a picture of an actress who knows how to seduce and radiate, and place it near where you get dressed every day. Rent movies that she stars in. Pause in the scenes where she "turns on her brights." Notice exactly how she does this, feel the process in your own body, and practice it!
- Get monthly mani-pedis. Let your brightly colored nails express the splendor of your embodied light.
- Go out of your way to wear sacred adornment every day — beautiful jewelry, makeup, scarves, shoes, handbags. Dress the part of a goddess, whatever that means for you.

Stepping into Your Golden Shadow

Our Golden Shadows are our brightest, most expansive qualities that went into hiding because we were reprimanded for expressing them as young children. We toned them down and settled into a ho-hum mediocrity so we wouldn't make other people feel uncomfortable. As a result, we live in a time where we're more afraid of our wonderfulness than we are of our awfulness; and, as we've seen, it's an arduous journey home to the joy and power that are our birthright.

Yes, feeling good and internalizing our heroes and heroines *is* hard work. Carl Jung, the man who gave language to the concept of the shadow, also suggested that it was often more difficult for people to get the gold out of their shadows than to get the skeletons out of their closets. As we've discussed, from an early age most of us learned to survive our childhoods by shutting down. We experienced sadness and anger while excluding the best parts of life. Consequently, we may find that when we finally start to experience more abundance, love, power, and pleasure as adult women, the surge in positive feelings can feel incredibly scary and threatening.

In fact, oftentimes as we stand at the threshold of realizing greater levels of success than we've ever known before, we self-sabotage ourselves. We get a cold before our big presentations. Our backs go out right after we get promotions, or we start to bicker with our fiancés right before we say "I do." We all have a certain set point for how much energy we can stand — at either end of the spectrum. We hold deeply ingrained patterns of constriction, and evolving requires that we systematically train ourselves to feel higher and higher highs, while also sustaining compassionate presence during our lowest of lows.

It's also important to recognize that our own set points are often directly related to our mothers' upper limits. What was the maximum amount of pleasure she was willing and capable of experiencing and receiving? It's up to each of us to hold the pinnacle of our lineages *and* pay our openness forward. Since we carry the unhealed wounds of our female lineage in our bodies and souls, the inner work we do has the power to heal through the generations. The ecstasy you open in your own body now will benefit the generations of women both before *and* after you.

Internalize Your Idols

In chapter 5, we explored how we project our own negative qualities onto someone else. Now it's time to take the opposite approach and own our projections so we can use them in a positive way.

First, write down your heroes and heroines. Under each name, list the qualities that you admire about that person. Then step back and look at the attributes. These are the elements of your Golden Shadow you need to assimilate.

On the last day of the retreats I lead, I warn women of what I call "the rubber band effect." It's something we all experience when we go home after a transformative week together. We've stretched our capacity, holding an unfamiliar, heightened experience of openness, happiness, and freedom in our bodies. When we jump back into our daily grind, it's hard to maintain this expansion. Maybe our loved ones feel threatened by our newfound power, or we dive back into unresolved conflict and revert to habitual defense mechanisms. Like rubber bands, we sharply snap back, contracting to a place of even *more* closure than was our norm *before* we went on retreat! This is okay. In fact, it's how we find our *new* normal. Soon enough we'll settle back to a sweet spot right smack in the middle — between the old, familiar closure and the fresh taste of radical opening. There we'll stay until we feel safe enough to once again shift our set point to experience even more goodness. This is how we evolve.

Whenever we seek transformation, we need to be sure we're ready to actually *receive* the abundance that awaits us on the other side. If we don't know how to let it in, we'll miss out on the fruits of our hard work. Ask yourself regularly, "How good can I stand it?" Test yourself with how much energy — both dark and light — you can handle in your system. Get familiar with how you contract, as well as with how you expand. What do both of these look like from the outside? How do they feel in your body? Continually strengthen your ability to receive *more*.

Grandeur is not just for celebrities or those who are "more fortunate." Greatness is your destiny too. This doesn't mean that you need to be rich and famous. It means that you deserve to be wildly happy, fulfilled, and turned on by life — in the ways that have the most heart and meaning for *you*. You have the unlimited power of the Goddess within you right now. Will you partner with this inner power? Untying and teasing out our repressed nobility is essential on our paths and must not be regarded as egotistical, "unspiritual," divergent sidetracks. In addition to being warriors who courageously explore the cracks of our unconscious, let's also be divas, feasting on our own deliciousness, drunk on our own fabulousness.

Jealousy: An Unexpected Detour to Greatness

Women who identify themselves as spiritual tend to have a very hard time admitting to themselves that they are jealous, especially of another woman's success, beauty, or power. When jealousy arises, it tends to go underground, and every single woman has experienced the result of this suppression. When women bury their feelings of jealousy, they succumb to the high school mean-girl syndrome, backstabbing, back-talking, or becoming queens of catty competition. Let's own it, sisters: we are very competitive with one another!

You need to grow up this part of yourself and use jealousy as an indication of where you're not living out your own dreams. Jealousy is never about *her*. It's always about *you*. Jealousy, like everything else that you feel or experience, is 100 percent your responsibility.

Six Steps to Turn Jealousy into Personal Power

1. Locate it in your body. When you first feel the jealousy, unhook the sensation from a story about "why" you're jealous. Find the feeling in your body. Where is it exactly? What does it feel like? What is its temperature, texture, and color?

2. Contact the sensation directly. Once you've located it, feel the sensation fully. Touch it directly with your heartfelt awareness. What is it like to step right inside the nucleus of the sensation and to let the feeling be as big as it needs and wants to be, without turning away?

3. Find your unbridled praise for the object of your jealousy and the unique flavor of the feminine that she lives and expresses. Later on, within the next twenty-four hours, reflect on what exactly about that other woman you are jealous of. Appreciate her for being your mirror, for holding the medicine of where you are holding back or longing for growth and expression. Do not continue onto the last step until you have fully found your praise for her. She represents a part of your own relationship with the feminine that needs healing.

4. Try her on in a low-risk scenario. In the shower, in your kitchen, or somewhere when the stakes aren't high, breathe her flavor of feminine finesse into your heart and belly. Move as she moves. Talk as she talks. Express as she expresses. Later, in public settings, if you feel emotionally triggered by her, keep trying her on, even though you will feel awkward, uncertain, and maybe even a little bit embarrassed. This is a sign that your nervous system is growing to hold her spectrum of energy. Keep going.

5. Praise her directly. Instead of backstabbing, if she's doing something that totally rocks and that gets your panties all in a bunch about it, appreciate her. Publicly. Send her an email. Text her. Post on her Facebook wall. And only praise, no passive-aggressive attacks of praise cloaked as criticism ("Great job! I thought *most* of the presentation was fantastic!"). Cheer her on. Let her know that what she's doing is totally awesome and how it inspires you.

6. Live in integrity. Don't flirt with her man. Don't woo her clients. Don't brush her off. Respect her. Celebrate her. Love her and the life that she has cultivated. Use her as an inspiration and a springboard into taking ownership for creating the life *you* most long for.

Nuggets of Gold

Shame, anger, sadness, fear, and vulnerability: these were some of the hard-to-face feelings that we turned to in the underworld. Now it's time to meet their bright counterparts like joy, desire, humor, pleasure, and wildness. These are equally hard for us to experience, because each holds disowned dimensions of our Golden Shadows. The noblest aspects of ourselves, they are often indicators of our highest callings, holding the keys to who we truly are and the unique gifts we're meant to share with the world.

It's important to note that as you resurrect these, you may feel some grief for only half-living portions of your life. Allow those feelings to flow too. What matters now is that you learn your lessons from the past and choose a new present based on the resulting wisdom. Devoid of self-condemnation, we can start anew in any moment.

You can work with any of these expansive feelings as you worked with your inner selves in chapter 6. Each of these is also a "voice" of the self. Remember, these important parts of ourselves will become our demons if they remain ignored and abused, and they will use their dark sister counterparts to get our attention through crisis. Let's give them our respect and attention instead.

Here are some ways to approach feelings such as joy, desire, humor, pleasure, and wildness.

Connecting with Expansive Feelings

For each of the following feelings, and any others you want to explore, ask yourself the following questions:

- Where do you feel this in your body?
- Which inner self or selves protects this feeling?
- When you dialogue directly with this, what does he or she have to say?

Joy: Joy exists independent of our moods or outer circumstances. Innocent giddiness and delight in being alive, joy is ebullient and unapologetic — even if those around us are down in the dumps. However, because of its effusiveness, joy can also feel incredibly threatening. As Brené Brown writes,

In a culture of deep scarcity — of never feeling safe, certain, and sure enough — joy can feel like a setup. We wake in the morning and think, *Work is going well. Everyone in the family is healthy. No major crises are happening. The house is still standing. I'm working out and feeling good. Oh, shit. This is bad. This is really bad. Disaster must be lurking right around the corner.*[2]

The higher you feel, the further the fall on the other side could be. This makes joy potentially the most difficult emotion to feel. To let more joy in, you need to recognize when it's there and practice opening to it, bodily. What, where, and who brings you the most joy? What about letting more joy in feels scary for you? How do you share your joy with others?

Desire: Neither selfish nor insignificant, our desires are the language of longing from our SHEs. Heeding them is a requirement for manifesting our deepest, clearest intentions. Since we all learned to cut ourselves off from our desires as little girls, it can be a long road back to reclaiming them. We need to start out small. During inconsequential moments of the day (e.g., making lunch, picking out an outfit, practicing a yoga pose), we need to ask, "What do I want right now?" Then we need to be good mothers to ourselves by giving ourselves what we desire. After doing this for a while, when faced with larger life decisions, we're more prepared. In those moments we can ask, "What do I really, truly want here, regardless of what other people think?"

Humor: We need to be careful that we don't get *too* serious in our pursuits of wisdom. The most enlightened people I know also have great senses of humor. We need to remember to laugh, have fun, and hold everything — especially ourselves — lightly. In a deck of cards, it's the "Joker" that's the wild card, able to be anything it wants to be. In ancient times, it was only the jester who could make fun of the king and queen without losing his head. When we stay loose and open and keep (or grow!) our sense of humor, we too can have this flexibility to morph and adapt ourselves and to break out of the trance of seriousness. What situations in your life might improve if you held things more lightly? What are a few ways you can play more this week?

Pleasure: Women wither under the tyranny of our stress hormones. Although we're often addicted to bemoaning the busyness of life, we flourish most in relaxation, with the secretion of feel-good hormones like oxytocin and serotonin. For us, pleasure is not a luxury, it's a necessity. Regena Thomashauer, author of *Mama Gena's School of Womanly Arts*, teaches "[When] your aim is pleasing yourself and having fun, success always follows."[3]

How did you see your mother or grandmother relate to pleasure? What truly, deeply nourishes you? What would it take for you to move closer toward those things? What would it look like for you to take 100 percent responsibility for your pleasure, not expecting anyone else to meet those needs?

Wildness: Dr. Clarissa Pinkola Estés, author of *Women Who Run with the Wolves*, writes, "Wildlife and the Wild Woman are both endangered species."[4] If you were to unleash your inner wild woman in your life — if you felt completely uninhibited and no one stood in your way — what would you do? What would that look like? What passions could be fueled by your willingness to let your wild woman out?

Also consider your relationships to beauty, play, abundance, compassion, adventure, gratitude, generosity, humility, peace, grace, and sovereignty.

Are there any other aspects of your Golden Shadow that you're ready to own and express?

The Art of Bragging

Many of us were raised with the belief that people who "showed off" were arrogant and boastful, so we didn't dare reveal our talents. As grown women we've probably learned to deflect praise and talk down what we've done to shift the focus off of us whenever we can. Or, conversely, perhaps we've tried to hog the spotlight. However, this is just another thwarted expression, springing from our confusion about our greatness.

When we constantly avoid being the center of attention, there's no way we can let the world know about the wondrous gifts we behold. Therefore, in addition to sharing our shame together, we need to also create a ritual for shamelessly "showing off."

Bragging Circle

One of the most adored women's circle practices I lead at the SHE Retreat is the Bragging Circle. During this counterpart to the Shame Circle, each woman grabs the talking stick and declares her sauciest, sexiest attributes and successes with the group.

Here's some of the gold that comes forth:

- I love my breasts, and I don't care that they sag. That's how I nourished my three beautiful children.
- I'm *super* organized. Give me any drawer, and I can organize the shit out of it.
- I'm an incredible poet. Give me any topic and I can write a poem about it that will move you to tears.
- Every man I've ever been with has told me I have a magic pussy. Apparently, it's quite something.
- I'm an *amazing* tango dancer. A real natural. I just seem to float across the floor.
- See this? This curve of my calf? My girlfriend always tells me how sexy this part of my leg is. I must say, I have to agree with her.
- I throw the best parties. I'm an amazing hostess!

If you held the talking stick right now, what would you brag about? Choose one to three things to shamelessly promote about your own greatness.

Divine Pride

Be not afraid of greatness: some are born great,
some achieve greatness, and some have greatness thrust upon 'em.

— William Shakespeare, *Twelfth Night*

I want to let you in on a little secret. But first, a celebration: When we bring both our Dark and Golden Shadows into consciousness, we experience a surge in self-esteem. This blossoms out of being honest with ourselves, honoring the beauty and power of our embodiment, authoring our own lives, and saying no to any more self-betrayal. Through these actions, we live in harmonious integrity with our SHEs and our outer realities. With increased self-esteem our health improves, mood uplifts, creativity surges, and relationships thrive.

Now for the secret. Self-esteem is relative. It ebbs and flows. Sometimes we feel confident; other times (*especially* when we're in transition) we don't. Rather than striving for self-esteem, we need to dig deeper. How do we keep striding toward our ascent, shining our light when we're feeling insecure? We need to understand that essence of who we all already, ultimately are.

From the perspective of Absolute reality, there's an even deeper layer of self-esteem that we need to palpate. It's called "Divine Pride," a concept I first learned from Ken Wilber. He defines this as

> a simple recognition of our holy heritage, and an acknowl-
> edgment of the tremendous responsibility that comes along
> with this recognition. This is not the braggadocio of a new
> age narcissist — it is a pride stripped of all arrogance, tem-
> pered by humility, and held with unwavering devotion to
> an intelligence infinitely greater than our own.[5]

Divine Pride reminds you that you were *already* born perfect. No wounding or failure could ever sully this. SHE lives within you, as you, allowing you to enjoy the full splendor of Her creation through your body — *always*. You can ignore, doubt, and forget this, but that doesn't change the indestructible truth that you already *are* this. Your presence alone, just as it is, feeds so many others in ways you could never fathom.

Deity Visualization Practice

Here's a practice from Tibetan Buddhism that returns us to Divine Pride by cultivating the certainty that we *are* god/goddess. It allows you to trust your inborn divine nature.

1. Look at an image of a deity — like a *thangka* (painting) or a *murti* (sculpture).
2. Take in as many details of the figure as you can through your vision and your memory.

3. Close your eyes and try to inwardly perceive and revive this image within your mind's eye.
4. Ultimately, with enough practice, grace enters and you *become* the deity. The I and the thou become one. From this recognition, Divine Pride emerges.

At the relative level, we *all* need this journey because we've forgotten who we truly are. But, at the Absolute level, you didn't need to embark on this journey to find the Divine Mother. You're already Her. You don't need to transcend your ego or even figure out what a soul is. SHE's already, always, the groundless ground of being, living within *all* of us, without exception. She's your closures and your openness, your thoughts and the space between your thoughts, your compulsions and your splendor. Rather than getting fixated on your limitations, honor Her by aiming your life in the direction of devotionally serving Her in your own imperfectly perfect way. Even during times when you fear your own innate greatness, don't hesitate a moment longer to activate the spark of the holy that resides within you.

Simply by reading this, you've become part of the solution to the world's pain. Snap out of your myopic obsessions with your shortcomings. Your false belief about your disconnection isn't serving anyone. No one ever has or will carry the same gift that you're here to share. Let this knowing be the beacon that guides your life. When you align your actions with your deepest devotion and purest intentions, they will be extensions of Her grace in a world that desperately needs it.

Journaling Questions

- What were the messages from your caretakers and teachers that caused you to shut down and feel ashamed about your Golden Shadow?
- How will you practice turning on your brights?
- How might a deeper recognition of your Divine Pride serve your life, and the world?

Chapter 11

Marrying the
Divine Masculine

*When you are able / to make two become one, / the inside like the outside /
and the outside like the inside / the higher like the lower, /
so that a man is no longer male, / and a woman, female, /
but male and female become a single whole… / then you shall enter in.*

— Gospel of Thomas

Take out a piece of paper and a pen. On the left side of the page, draw a circle. On the right side, draw another circle, making sure that the two circles overlap right in the center of the page, forming a crescent. Last, color in that crescent. Now, put your pen down, step back, and take a look.

This crescent is a *mandorla*, the Italian word for "almond." A simple model for how to grasp life's greatest paradoxes, the mandorla depicts the overlapping opposites we've been integrating within ourselves, and, on an even larger scale, between spirit and matter in the fertile overlay of our SHEs. Rather than boxing things into "either/or" categories, we can use the mandorla to instead see them through the lens of "both/and." In this single image, the tension of the opposites ease, and life's sometimes painfully perplexing opposites find a unifying ground.

We've already reconciled *a lot* of opposites on our journey thus far. Now that we're nearing the end of our Heroine's Journey, before our final celebratory homecoming can transpire, we have one last *big* shift we *have* to make. It's a shift that's frequently overlooked in conversations about the Divine Feminine, but its omission would leave us forever incomplete. We've explored our relationships with our mothers, the Divine Mother, the Patriarchy, our Inner Patriarchs, demons, and daemons. We've seen how we're Father's Daughters. But we have yet to fully explore our relationships with our fathers and the Divine Masculine.

Perhaps even more than the Divine Feminine, the Divine Masculine lives in shadow. Very few of us have any idea what He looks or feels like. It's time for you to discover this directly, because in order to be a whole, powerful women, you must heal your Inner Divine Masculine to serve, partner with, and protect your SHE. A Heroine only arrives at her homecoming *after* she has integrated the HE into the mandorla of her SHE.

The Divine Masculine vs. the Inner Patriarch

As we explored earlier, in the West women are starting to become the family breadwinners, excelling in traditionally masculine arenas like politics and business, but we have largely had to become pseudo-males, sacrificing our femininity, to do so. Likewise, more and more men are embracing the feminine domains of being stay-at-home fathers and focusing on relationships, sacrificing their masculinity. Switching roles isn't the answer; finding the harmony of the mandorla *within* and *between* each of these roles is.

What's needed at this time for real healing is the full reclamation and harmonization of both Divine Feminine *and* Divine Masculine qualities. Fortunately, the archetype for this potential already exists in the world's most sacred cultures. The ancient Indian Shiva *Lingam* offers a symbolic representation of this human and cosmic potential. It depicts the phallus, or the male principle of creation, *Shiva*, both cradled by and penetrating the yoni, or the female principle of creation, *Shakti*. The ancient Taoist symbol of yin and yang also depicts this commingling unity. Masculine and feminine can complement, support, and complete — rather than *compete* with — each other.

We have a ways to go before fully living this realization. As is true for everything on this path, the first step is recognition. We have to directly *see* and *acknowledge* how the masculine principle operates within our own psyches and what kind of effect that has on our lives. For example, when women begin working with me, most come feeling run down and depleted (quintessential Father's Daughters). "My masculine is just fine," they say. "In fact, he's *too* good at what he does! What can I do to strengthen my relationship with my feminine?" Such women — and I can only say this because I've been there too — are not at all "fine" with their masculine. In fact, I have rarely met a woman *anywhere* who truly is.

What we mistake as "fine" is our unconscious submission to our inner Pushers, Perfectionists, Controllers, and Critics — or our Inner Patriarchs. What most of us consider to be "masculine" is the deranged, patriarchal masculine — one that is equally damaging to men and women. We mistake the Inner Patriarch for the Divine Masculine. The former shoves, drives, and forces us to exert beyond our body's instincts, overriding our innate rhythms, pleasure, and desires. He's what brings us to women's work in the first place! In this way, we come here believing that the "masculine" is the problem and the answer is to completely shun this part of ourselves by focusing only on our "feminine."

If we end here, focusing solely on women, our journeys are incomplete. Since we all have inner "masculine" and "feminine," yin and yang energies, believing that our final destiny is to usurp the Patriarchy and to replace it with strictly feminine principles denies us of the power that surges forth when we activate and unite both of these essential facets of ourselves. The consequences of being out of touch with your Divine Masculine can be quite severe.

Here are some signs that your Divine Masculine is in shadow:

- You're unable to set and maintain clear boundaries.
- You suffer from either repressed anger (a lot of shame) or you erupt in toxic, volcanic rage.
- You suffer from a lack of self-discipline and are unable to follow through on your goals and dreams from start to finish.

- You have a weak ego (resulting in a strong Inner Critic, Inner Patriarch, etc.).
- You feel hypersensitive and carry within you a very volatile, vulnerable child.
- You experience crippling emotions that prevent you from consistently showing up for your life.
- You identify with being a victim and don't know how to face your challenges as a warrior.
- Your creativity feels dried up or nonexistent.
- You're in a constant battle for control with your body.
- You tend to manipulate others to get what you want.
- You fear true intimacy.
- You often feel exhausted, depleted, and overwhelmed.
- You're a workaholic and your life is out of balance.
- You stay in abusive relationships.
- You're unable to earn, save, or manage your money.
- You're disorganized and often running late.
- Your actions don't line up with your core values.
- You procrastinate.
- You feel confused about or disconnected from your life purpose.

Do you see the grave consequences of excluding the Divine Masculine from your life? Now that we understand that He *isn't* your Inner Patriarch, let's get crystal clear on who, exactly, He *is*, because if you want your SHE to thrive in the world, you must activate the disowned self whose sacred duty it is to protect and serve Her.

Who Is the Divine Masculine?

Along with two images of the Divine Feminine, my altar also houses two images of the Divine Masculine: the Buddha and Archangel Michael. The Buddha's steadfast, seated meditation posture reminds me to stay rooted like a mountain amid life's storms. A container of spacious stillness holds and sustains my vulnerable core. Archangel Michael's sword of discernment can slice through any situation — no matter how sticky or complex — with skillful means. His shield protects me from harm, and his purple cape allows him to show up, in service of anyone who needs him, at a moment's notice. Just as the Buddha's equanimity has no limits, Archangel Michael's service has no end, so long as they both stay rooted in honoring the highest truth in every moment.

When you are in touch with Him, you can protect yourself against your Inner Patriarch and provide a safe harbor for your Inner Little Girl. You can serve and enact the deep desires and longings of your SHE. You can speak up, either to deactivate your dominant inner selves or to call forth the wisdom from your disowned selves. Your Inner Divine Masculine helps to lead your inner family. He's a rightful comaster of your inner household, right alongside your SHE. That's a really important, powerful position in your psyche! Let's take some time to get to know Him better. Here are some qualities of the Divine Masculine, inner *and* outer:

- Communicates His needs clearly and compassionately, even if they may initially evoke conflict
- Sets boundaries, but not barriers
- Exerts His willpower and self-discipline as a means to realize His deepest longings and core values
- Feels His heart without overindulging His feelings
- Doesn't collapse into others' agendas
- Never, ever turns away from His truth
- Creates the necessary structures and containers to actualize His purpose (in money, work, family, spiritual practice, relationships, health, etc.)
- Penetrates every moment fully with His direct, yet spacious, presence
- Witnesses thoughts and feelings
- Makes clear, assertive decisions
- Serves selflessly
- Fiercely and loyally protects, provides for, and serves what and whom He most loves
- Remains courageous and imperturbable in the face of challenges
- Takes consistent action arising from an integrated understanding of His intellect and intuition
- Exerts His power without force or manipulation

Support and Challenge

Here are three simple ways to dip your toes into your *life-affirming* masculine energy, without throwing your SHE overboard. The healthy masculine thrives when he feels both challenged *and* supported. See how these activities encourage you to grow your capacity *through* embracing challenge. As we explored with our SHE Cycles, we all need regular doses of adversity to strengthen the warrior ethos within our own bodies and psyches. Luckily, life already serves up plenty of opportunities to practice this!

1. Small challenge: Right now, feel your spine. Feel the bright, white saber of clarity that *is* the backbone of your body — and your life. As you inhale, feel your breath traveling down the front surface of your spine. As you exhale, feel it riding up the back of your spine, from your tailbone to the crown of your head. Experience how your spine offers support to the vulnerable front surface of your body. Explore how you can more deeply relax and surrender around the support of your spine.

2. Medium challenge: Commit to a mindfulness meditation practice — at the same time and place (consistency is key!) every day for a month. Set a timer for fifteen minutes (beginner) or thirty minutes (intermediate), shifting your position as needed within the first minute to make sure you're comfortable. After that, do not move for *any* reason. Don't scratch an itch. Don't fix your hair or take off your sweater. Don't look out the window if you hear the doorbell ring. Concentrate on the fluctuation of breath in your belly center. Acknowledge thoughts, feelings, stimuli, and sensations as they arise; yet remain unwavering in your concentration amid the incessant change within and around you.

3. Bigger challenge: On alternate days of the week, opt for more yang-enhancing embodiment practices like cardio, weight lifting, and flow yoga. The aim here is to build heat, increase endurance, and grow muscle mass. (Then on the days in between, choose more yin-enhancing embodiment practices like yin or restorative yoga, walks in nature, or flowing dance classes.) The key is to not take these on as a means of pushing or punishing yourself. Intention is everything. Allow these to instead flow from your desire to be a strong, resilient woman. I personally love being able to lift heavy objects or hike a mountain without huffing and puffing. Strong is sexy!

For those of you who are shaking your heads and waving your fists saying, "Noooo! I'm not ready for this! It has felt so juicy, good, and loooong overdue to coax my SHE out of the dark. My inner feminine is just now starting to shine!" I hear you. Yes, please, *do* honor where you are. Fully. Remember, we're all embracing our own rhythms as we move through this journey. If you're not ready for this, pause, work with the preceding materials for as long as you need to, and come back to this chapter when you feel ready.

If it's resistance you feel more than a lack of readiness, ease into this gradually. You don't need to do all the exercises. Just start with one or two that feel the most accessible. Incorporate more over time. It's perfectly understandable that you might arrive here and feel afraid that your Inner Masculine will dominate your SHE. Remember, yang energy dominates yin by its very nature. You need to feel very strong in your yin energy, and to have the capacity to both perceive and cultivate it, before you can find a harmonious inner dance between the two. This is lifelong learning!

Wherever you currently land in the spectrum of readiness to embrace your inner He, know this: every woman needs to become her own Prince Charming! Take time to dialogue with Him. What's His name? What does He look like? What messages does He have for you? This relationship is yours to cultivate.

Here's how one of the women in the SHE School visualized the relationship between her SHE and her Inner Divine Masculine:

> I am beginning to see an image of a Divine Masculine in
> this moment that mirrors my SHE. I realize that it has
> been there all along. My SHE always sits in a seated pos-
> ture at the base of a beautiful, tall tree and in this moment
> I see that tree shape shifting into a tall masculine form in
> a robe and then back into the tree.

As this vision reflects, however He shows up for you, your Inner Divine Masculine *wants* to serve you. He wants you to feel safe to be vulnerable, express yourself freely and creatively, and sculpt your entire life around your deepest longings. He's ready for you to call out to Him for help and guidance. Waiting in the wings, He's the part of your own psyche that knows how to solve problems, fix things, and build structures to support your vision. He wants to swoop in and help you clear the time and space you need to focus on what you love, stay aligned with your goals and inner guidance, cultivate your will to follow through amid life's storms, and find true and lasting success on your path. Even if you've never met a man (or woman who identifies more with the masculine principle) who offers you all these things, remember that we all already hold Him within us. We just need to learn to uncover and activate Him.

Mother Love and Father Love

We have already looked at cultivating a healthy inner Mother Love, or feminine compassion, for holding all of our inner selves in an embrace of unconditional love. Now we need to cultivate a healthy inner Father Love, or masculine compassion, to encourage us to grow and take action in the world — despite our fears and vulnerabilities.

Sarah Powers, in her book *Insight Yoga*, further explains these concepts, which she drew from philosopher Ken Wilber:

> Mother love promotes willing acceptance, while father love develops inspiration toward improvement.... Mother love is connected to beingness; father love is aligned with evolution. Mother love lets us value ourselves and others just as we are, whereas father love knows there is always more to learn and room for change.... Ultimately we need both in healthy doses to grow into sane and functional adults who are able to experience authentic intimacy. When we have divorced these essential attributes, it is like hopping around on one foot — we are easily thrown off balance by the slightest challenge.[1]

If we activate only feminine compassion, we collapse into a pathologically yin disposition. In a meditation practice, this looks like squirming in your seat, ceaseless fidgeting, identifying with every thought and feeling, and being unable to follow through on your initial intention and commitment to practice. If we activate only masculine compassion, we're bullied by a pathologically yang temperament. A meditation practice enacted from that place looks like rigidly holding your posture even if you're in pain and risking injury, slicing out any and all feelings from your awareness, striving and competing with yourself or others, and closing your heart.

When Mother and Father Love operate together, they form the two coessential wings of inner support that comprise attunement — contact and space — that we need to be fully functioning human beings. Feminine compassion makes loving contact. Masculine compassion offers space. In a meditation practice this looks like staying elegant and steady in your position, witnessing everything that arises in and around you with an intimate embrace of loving-kindness. Meditation then becomes the discipline of not turning away, married to the devotion of compassionately embracing everything you're facing. You meet whatever arises with both the grace of a sovereign queen and the nobility of a warrior king.

Within daily life, you can call upon masculine compassion to speak the hard truths of life when they're in service of another's highest good. You might need to tell a childhood friend that you haven't felt met by your friendship in a long while and it's time for your relationship to change. It could be time to talk to your parents about what plans they have in place for their old age and deaths. Maybe it's time to confront your partner about an addiction that's been the elephant in the living room for far too long.

This works internally too. Sometimes we need to unleash masculine compassion on *ourselves*. Is it time to call bullshit on how much time you're spending on the Internet when what you really want is to produce your own film? Do you evade your morning and evening rituals, feeling overwhelmed and scattered as a result? Do you keep eating a food that you know makes you feel awful? Call upon Him to help you knock it off — not because He wants to brutishly "keep you in line," but because He deeply *cares*.

Masculine compassion can seem ruthless at times in its action, like tough love, except it always comes fiercely from the heart and roots for the other person's success. Get to know it. Explore little ways every day that you can exercise this muscle, further strengthening your inner warrior. Every powerful woman needs to have a working relationship with her own masculine compassion. It's the key to creating the containers that we need in order to grow our dreams and to enact the boundaries that will protect them.

Forgiving Your Father

You knew this was coming! Copiloting life with our Inner Divine Masculine only transpires when we're able to forgive our fathers (and father figures if our biological fathers didn't help raise us). At their root, they are one and the same. You will never manifest the true love of your He (inner *or* outer) without first forgiving your father. Forgiveness resides at the heart of every spiritual practice. It opens us to loving without conditions and releasing toxic resentments that keep us imprisoned in the illusion of our separateness.

Here are some healing inquiries to help you get there, which I've drawn from a transformational retreat that I attended several years ago called the Hoffman Process, designed to liberate us from our childhood programming. This approach involves four stages:

1. Finding understanding without condemnation for your parents
2. Finding compassion for the childhood you've lived
3. Finding forgiveness for what your parents did to you and what you did to them
4. Finding total acceptance of them for who and what they were and are[2]

I know this can be a lot to ask, especially if you had an unsavory experience with your father figure growing up. This is a process. Be very gentle with yourself. Here are the steps to begin. You can write down your responses in your journal.

- What was it like for you to live in your childhood home with your father? Write a paragraph about this from the perspective of your eight-year-old self (speaking in the first person and present tense).
- What was the father of your childhood like (personality, behavior, etc.)?
- What negative patterns, moods, and attitudes did your father enact during your childhood?
- Look over the list of your father's negative patterns. Circle all of the

ones that you have adopted (past or present). Draw a star next to each one you've rebelled against by embracing its opposite.

- Next to each of the negative patterns that you've adopted, write down what the positive alternative is.
- Use your imagination to interview your father's Vulnerable Child. Ask his Inner Little Boy what it was like to be him, growing up in the way he did. Write this all down. Next, conduct an imaginary interview in your journal with your father — either as he is now or as you remember him. Ask him whatever you want to know about why he did what he did, and why he is who he is.
- Write a letter to your father, letting him know all the ways he hurt you and what you still resent him for. Then curse and scream as you violently rip it up and burn it.
- Write a letter to your father, letting him know all the things you appreciate about him. Recall as many positive memories of him as you can. If he's still alive, send it to him.

Note: If you want, you can go back to chapter 2 and repeat these same steps for your mother.

Remember, our psyches can't tell the difference between ritual and real life! Seemingly simple exercises like this can profoundly shift your relationships and free you from some outdated programming into more of an authentic, individuated life.

Boundaries: I Am. You Are.

I sat in a chair, my feet flat on the floor. The healer asked me to stretch my arms out to the sides with my palms facing down.

"We're going to do some muscle testing," she announced.

Several taps, presses, and pokes later, she interrupted, "Hold on just a minute. Let me go get something."

She scurried behind me, where I could hear her rustling through papers.

"Aha, here it is!" she exclaimed. Then she returned to stand in front of me.

"This is an important message for you, from the Divine Feminine," she announced, waving the paper in the air.

I sat up a little straighter. *Okay*, I told myself, *I thought I was coming for craniosacral therapy, but I'll take this too.*

"You need better boundaries. You take in too much from other people because you're so sensitive. What you came here for today isn't yours. It's other people's stuff. I'll help you clear it, and then I'll teach you how to clear it yourself going forward. In order for you to be a truly powerful healer, you need to understand this concept." She inhaled, leaving us both inside a pregnant pause.

"Here's the message," she continued. "I am. You are."

I am. You are. I repeated silently to myself.

"Whenever you are around others and you start to feel their energy coming into you, say that to yourself."

I am. You are.

Sisters, hold on to this mantra and use it often. The Divine Masculine superpower of boundary setting consistently shows up as one of our biggest challenges. Either we don't set them and then overextend ourselves because we want to be good girls, or we revolt and go the other way and create *rigid barriers* — keeping nourishment of all varieties at bay. Every boundary needs to be like a porous cell membrane that sometimes expands and sometimes contracts, all the while letting positive nutrients in and wastes out.

Clear Your Energy Body

The more you fill up your own energy field, the less work you need to do defending your boundaries. You can practice this in the shower, in bed, or on your meditation cushion (anywhere!). It helps you to make sure you're filling yourself up with the energy of your own soul rather than taking on what's not yours.

- Extend your arms straight out from your sides. This is the span of your own energy body. It extends in all directions.
- Sense this energy field, and trust whatever you notice about it. You

do this naturally every time you talk to someone. Notice how when some people get too close you instinctually step back a little so they don't step into your energy field. With others it might feel okay for this kind of energetic intimacy.

- Just as you adjust your energy field with other people, you can adjust it within yourself. When you're at home or in a serene place in nature, it might feel better to have a wider energy field that's farther away from your body and more porous to the external world. When you're in an airplane or a busy mall, you'll want to pull your energy field in closer to you and make its edges more firm, to keep the cacophonous external energy from entering.
- To heal and strengthen your energy field as a protective force around you, visualize it as a golden-pink light.
- At the end of each day, call your own energy back. In whatever ways you've been extending yourself, intentionally bring it back inside your energy field. Likewise, consciously release any energy that is not yours: "I call my energy back from all of my activities and interactions today. I release any energies that are not mine, and I allow my soul to be the clearest, strongest energy in my body, my energy field, and my life."

To define the boundary between "I" and "You," call on your Inner Divine Masculine. Ask Him to take out His sword and slice through what is no longer necessary for you to be carrying. Just because your girlfriend is in a bad mood doesn't mean that you need to be. Just because your brother is going through a crisis doesn't mean that you need to downplay your win. In fact, the best gift you can ever give anyone who's going through a hard time is to keep your vibration high and your energy strong. You must keep the joy flowing. You can still have empathy when you're in a good mood. We're all on different growth tracks. Be on yours and let others be on theirs.

Feel how cutting things away opens up so much new space and potential. Use your Inner Divine Masculine to clarify your yeses and nos. Dialogue with your Inner Little Girl to see what she needs so He can protect her from now on. Identify the areas in your life where you're afraid to speak your needs because you feel guilty and fear they'll cause conflict. *I am. You are.* Notice how repressing these needs harms you *and* the other. When you try to manage someone else's reaction, you leave zero room for finding a creative solution to the problem because you have such a tight grip on it.

After a month of exploring her relationship with her Inner Masculine, one of the sisters in our SHE School shared the following:

> People respond pretty well when boundaries are clear. My pleaser told me people would be upset with me. But I realized that when I use my Divine Masculine to speak my truth, they may not be happy about them from the outset, but they respect them. I feel like my boss actually respects me more after setting a boundary and clearly communicating my needs.

When you take steps to set your boundaries for others, be ready for things to be messy. The other person may get angry. You may risk either ending or changing the relationship. Let yourself off the hook from needing to do it perfectly. (You won't. That's not the point) Accept the consequences.

Also, it's highly likely that you'll have a big Inner Critic attack after setting a new boundary. Be prepared to dialogue with your inner selves to clean up the aftermath. But, at the end of the day, ask yourself this: Would I rather be comfortable or tell the truth? Choose freedom. Always. Choose ending the self-defeating pattern of falling asleep to your own needs. If it's coming from your heart, that truth will always serve the highest intention in you and others.

Explore Your Boundaries

- What are you taking on that's not yours to carry?
- What are you letting in that needs to be kept out?
- Who would you be if you stood your own ground?
- What feels uncomfortable about being joyful when another is suffering? Is there a way to hold joy within yourself and compassion for the other simultaneously?

- Where and with whom do you feel challenged in speaking your truth and creating firm, yet flexible, boundaries?
- What needs are you afraid to own and protect?
- What impact do your loosey-goosey or too-tight boundaries have on you? On others?

Hieros Gamos: The Sacred Marriage

Keith and I have a relationship altar in our bedroom. In its center resides a brass Buddhist statue known as Yab-Yum, which literally means "father-mother" in Tibetan. The male deity sits in a meditation posture, while the female deity straddles him, entwining her arms and legs around his back, throwing her head back in rapture. This depicts the ecstatic union between masculine and feminine — two halves of a whole, integrated human being. It illustrates how the subtle energy of the Divine Masculine and Feminine join together within our own bodies. The feminine moves in wide, concentric spirals around our midline. The masculine extends linearly, along the vertical access of our spines. When we learn to conduct these energies in our bodies, psyches, and lives, we experience the sacred marriage of this inner "twosome," which, when expressed through partnership at the outer level, is truly a "foursome," for each has already realized the sacred marriage within *themselves*. They don't *need* each other for completion or wholeness. They unite out of a conscious choice to together uphold the regeneration of life through and as their love.

We can never know such true love without first celebrating this divine union within. This Sacred Marriage, or *hieros gamos*, *is* the mandorla. The place where opposites unite, where the lower self marries the higher Self. The masculine marries the feminine. The yin unites with the yang, the inner with the outer. The Sacred Marriage stands at the conclusion of nature's cycles, at the threshold of spring's promise of regeneration and renaissance. Likewise, when a woman marries her True Self, she has honestly lived and learned from each season. Through the ripening of her inner wisdom, she is truly ready to give birth to her new life.

Wed Your True Self

Rituals prepare us for new life. Create a simple ceremony to honor this union within yourself and to prepare for crossing the threshold into your rebirth. Your ritual doesn't need to be anything fancy. Simple is powerful! Feel free to incorporate some of these ideas or to create your own:

- Write vows to yourself, communicating ways that you will uphold the wisdom you've acquired.
- Buy yourself a ring or another symbol of your union.
- Purify your sacred space. Light candles, burn sage, play music, buy flowers, and rearrange your altar. Add movement, prayer, or whatever other elements feel right for you.
- Go on retreat or to a beautiful place in nature. Take time for yourself to journal and integrate this commitment to your Self.
- Prepare a beautiful meal and share it with those you love.

As a sisterhood, we'll all move into the next stage of our journey together. See and feel yourself crossing over a threshold as bride and bridegroom both, into your new life.

The Sovereign Virgin

On the other side of this threshold awaits yet another archetype on our journey, the Virgin: she who's impregnated with your new life. In Tibetan sacred iconography, the Dakini depicts this archetype when she holds her *khaṭvāṅga*, or staff, in one hand. This symbolizes her Inner Divine Masculine. It's the representation of the fierce clarity of Father Love that she has learned to integrate in order to Awaken.[3]

When a woman holds her own *khaṭvāṅga* and resides in the mandorla, she has fully passed through all three of the Triple Goddess archetypes of the relative realm (Maiden, Mother, and Crone) and transcended them to become a Virgin — the Divine Feminine archetype that exists *beyond* life's seasons and cycles. The Virgin is a woman who has dedicated her life to protecting and nourishing divine love.

Marion Woodman describes the Virgin not as a sexually untouched woman, as most of us have come to understand the term *virgin*, but more like a native forest or a stretch of untainted wilderness.[4] Like Virgin Mary, impregnated with divine love, the Virgin archetype is whole, belonging to Herself, and open to all of life. Through Her inner work, the conscious Virgin is "she who is who she is because that is who she is."[5]

Because the Virgin reconciles all opposites within Her, like the Virgin Mother she has everything she needs inside of Her to create new life. Fully in touch with Her inner resources, She can dynamically respond to life, activating the depth and breadth of Her faculties to serve humanity. In this way, the Virgin shows us that, as women, in order to fully give our gifts to the world we all need to operate from this disposition of integrated masculine and feminine energies, discovering a new, more fluid and genderless place that opens the portal to our greatest potential.

On this, innovative psychologist Mihaly Csikszentmihalyi writes, "Creative individuals are more likely to have not only the strengths of their own gender but those of the other one, too."[6] To actualize our gifts in the world, we need to find this place of inner androgyny. In some moments we focus, deeply penetrating a problem with our intellects. In other moments we open and soften, holding the problem without fixation. Spiritually, this androgyny exists as well. Each gender can travel different paths to Awakening, but we all, ultimately, arrive in the same place — in the ultimate freedom to live from our one true nature.

In my own life, while I'm deeply feminine in my core, when I'm teaching or writing I do become androgynous, able to flow and morph between genders in order to elicit whatever is most needed to serve and open a moment. I once judged myself about this, thinking that I "should" be more feminine *all* the time, but as I grow I embrace that I have a gift for navigating this complexity. I am able to do more for others (and myself) when I don't try to stuff myself into a single box. The less afraid we are of living in the paradox that sometimes we need to be more masculine to be more of a woman (or vice versa), the more the fertile possibility for a life of radical service opens before us.

Using Your Androgyny to Thrive

Each day, before you start a new activity, look at what needs to be done and determine what kind of energy you most need to draw on. If you're answering emails, call on your Divine Masculine to keep time and create strong, flexible boundaries. If you're cooking, call on your Divine Feminine to savor the smells, flavors, and sounds. When we consciously conduct our energy, we have ready access to the inner resources we need to meet the present moment at our fullest capacity.

This journey to sovereign Virginity awakens so many capacities within us that we previously didn't even know existed, and the result is not that we become more superhuman. We actually become more human, quirkier, more ordinary. More fully ourselves. We start being more at home in our foibles, less apologetic about our idiosyncrasies, and more candid. Through this, we bring both a humor and a deep sense of calm to every encounter. We understand how things are and who we are, and we don't get hung up on wanting things to be otherwise.

True intimacy — with yourself, your higher purpose, or your beloved — is not possible until you arrive in this essential independence from all roles and bonds, into your own deep sense of living as your essence.[7] When the Virgin archetype takes root in you, your cells literally begin to vibrate at a new frequency. The experience of this integrated power moving into your physical body is unmistakable, and it's a sign that your initiation is now taking root at the deepest, densest level of your being.

From this stance, you know who you are and what you truly want. You are able to make your own empowered choices, independent and finally free of your mother and father, free of the dictates of your conditioning and acculturation. You are able to see beyond your myopic, egoic agendas in order to act for the benefit of all. You fully inhabit your inner home as a sovereign parent. Your life vision and transcendent inner voices are grounded in your heart and belly. You are ripe with your own potential, pregnant with your devoted integrity and authenticity.

Journaling Questions

- Where do you see the Divine Masculine in the world? In yourself?
- What areas in your life need more Father Love? What actions do you need to take to express this?
- Do you know any Virgins? What can you learn from them?
- Explore ways that you can use the androgyny of your inner Sacred Marriage to help you more creatively and efficiently achieve your goals and dreams.

Chapter 12

Birthing Your
Beautiful Life

What we play is life.

—Louis Armstrong,
Louis Armstrong, in His Own Words: Selected Writings

Muses come in many sizes and shapes. One of mine is nine years old and just happens to be the daughter of a pirate. She has bright red braids that stick out straight above her ears and striped knee socks that slouch inside clunky black boots. She doesn't give a hoot about being ladylike and funds her outlandish schemes with piles of gold and chests of hidden treasures. She lives alone in a rickety wooden house with a pet monkey, Mr. Nilsson. She's Pippi Longstocking, the leading lady in Swedish author Astrid Lindgren's classic book, published back in 1945, and now the feisty star of countless children's books, movies, and TV shows worldwide.

Along with millions of little girls everywhere, I held Pippi in the spotlight as one of my *most* cherished girlhood heroines. And, along with millions of women everywhere, as I grew up, I slowly forgot about her. She seemed, in my late teens and early twenties, an outgrown figment of a lost childhood, utterly unimportant next to my oh-so-serious adult concerns. That is, until 2010, right after I submitted the final manuscript for *The Way of the Happy Woman*, when we reconnected once more.

In Santa Fe, New Mexico, to attend a Transformational Speaking Intensive with my public speaking coach, Gail Larsen, I arrived expecting an "adult" course on PowerPoint presentations and poised professionalism. I brought my most serious adult expression, my most serious adult concerns, and my most serious adult problems to be solved. However, during my four days there, my serious shell slowly cracked when I reunited with two muses who resurfaced to show me the next steps on my path. The first was Mary Magdalene (as I wrote about at the start of the book), and the second was Pippi.

On the third afternoon of the intensive, we all sat outside on the inn's sun-drenched deck across from a partner. I snuggled up inside my big beige cotton sweater to warm myself from the autumn breeze and answered some questions. What is the story that most signifies why I do what I do? What are the qualities that I bring to my work? After sharing my responses, I received constructive feedback from my partner, a wise woman in her midsixties named Monique.

"You speak a lot from your little girl voice, up in your throat," she shared. "Bring it down here, into your belly. Like a woman," she instructed, pointing to the small bulge under her blouse. "You have a deep sensuality and sexiness, coupled with a playful innocence. I'd love to see you share more of these, intermingled together, when you speak."

Later that evening, we all took our partner's reflections back to our rooms to stew in. Our assignment: to extract from our feedback and personal experience what we believed to be our signature message, or what Gail, and the Shamanic teachings she draws from, calls our "original medicine." This is our own unique creative genius, or daemon, which we alone were born to bring into this world and which, if we don't, will be lost to the world forever.

Late that night, before I went to bed, my original medicine struck, like a bell ringing from within, as I drifted off to sleep:

The Tao of Queen Pippi.

"Oh my God! Yes! Yes! That's it!" I exclaimed as I leapt out of bed to scribble it down in my journal so I wouldn't forget it in the morning. The phrase unlocked for me the perfect reconciliation of my grown-up womanly grace, my love of nature's way, or the Tao, and my long-lost little girl pizzazz.

The next morning, when it was my turn to share my original medicine during my final presentation, I shed the layers of seriousness, inhibition, and self-consciousness that I'd been piling on since puberty. In doing so, I found Pippi again. Rambunctious, confident, and fun, she didn't bat an eye at public speaking. My Magical Little Girl had returned! On stage that morning, I realized that if I was ever going to fulfill what I identified as a huge part of my life purpose — public speaking — I needed my little Pippi to help. Why? Because she reminded me of lots of things: that the world was fresh and magical, that new experiences were fun, that failure didn't equal disaster, and that making new friends was the best part of it all. Wild and improper, she wasn't afraid to stand on a stage — she (I) had been a ballerina, after all!

Every woman needs to resurrect her own Pippi equivalent in her pursuits of feminine power. Connecting with your inner Pippi is just as important as communing with the gracefully gowned Goddess. With all of our ambitious to-dos and spiritual seeking, we also need to remember how to be messy, play, don our pigtails, eat with our fingers, wear rainbow-striped knee socks, be willing to say the wrong thing at the wrong time to the wrong person, and believe that *anything* is possible. Yes, of course, there's a time and a place to be prim and proper and to hunker down and exert some good old-fashioned discipline. But not at the expense of forgetting how to let that all go, send our Inner Critics off for a siesta, throw conventional notions of self-care out the window, and give ourselves permission to do *whatever* we darn please. At *any* age. *Silliness isn't just for little girls*. We women need it too! In fact, we're not really women at all when we're out of touch with the magic and endless optimism of our Inner Little Girls.

The Medicine of Your Magical Child

As a child, what activities did you get so absorbed in that you lost track of time? They harbor your invincible capacity to be joyously alive. Here we find, yet again, that to move forward in our lives, we have to travel backward. It's through journeying back to this whimsical, adolescent girl within each of us that we find the vitality and freshness we need to thrive in adulthood.

Even though it may take your entire life to fully return to this place of wondrous innocence and awe within, the reunion with your Magical Child is not to be missed. She's the sparkle in your daemon, and she emerges out of your Vulnerable Child when she feels held in the daily presence of your unconditional Mother Love *and* protective Father Love.

It's important to recognize that if she feels you're being cold and overly rational, she won't return. She needs to feel you lighten up to emerge. If you feel disconnected from this playful part of your SHE, it's time to make some changes to call her back.

With the return of the Magical Child, the Divine Child of Love — *your* Divine Child of Love — is born, carrying the seeds of your new life. Since trinities hold the sacred order of life, she's the third entity that is born from your inner union between the Divine Feminine and the Divine Masculine to complete the sacred triad.

The mysterious new life that has been trying to show itself now sees that, in the presence of our inner, unified love, it can use our very bodies and lives as its canvas. Through the act of creation resulting in this third entity, we all become Divine Mothers. We now know what it is to inhabit two worlds — the one in front of and behind the veil. We discover that, in order to regenerate life and access our true power, we need to be in this world but not of it. Like the Virgin Mother, we need to cocreate with our divinity as well as our humanity — with reverent nobility *and* playful levity.

From this place of creative, spontaneous play, life's greatest inventions emerge. Yet we all too frequently dismiss it as extravagant and unnecessary. *Who has time to play?* we ask. But if we *don't* take time to play, leaving stretches of unstructured time to dream, delight in life, and "be," our greatest ideas and creations will forever elude us.

How do you find your way back to this spontaneous, childlike nature? You need to journey back to your prepubescent self. Most likely, you lost her because you grew up too quickly. Perhaps you needed to take care of your own parents by being the good girl. Maybe you were told that you could only play or express your joy at certain times and in certain ways. To heal this, you don't need to force more play in your life. Resurrecting your relationship with your Magical Child will simply *bring* it to you. She's already within you, ready to playfully help you bring your SHE's gifts into the world.

Connect with Your Magical Child

Reflect on the following in your journal:

- What were your favorite ways to play as a child?
- Do you allow yourself to play as an adult? If so, how?
- How can you allow your grownup self to lighten up in new and interesting ways, every day?

Action Steps

- Schedule one "playdate" for yourself a week. Put it in your calendar. For example, you might go horseback riding, visit a botanical garden, attend a performance, enjoy a cupcake, make a new playlist, explore a funky shop, or take an art class.
- Dialogue with your Magical Child like you did with your Inner Critic and Vulnerable Child in chapter 6.
- Schedule (at least) two weeks of vacation time a year. If you can't afford to go away, plan a staycation. Add these to your calendar. Save and plan for them well in advance. Choose locales and activities that deeply nourish and inspire you.
- One hour a week, let your Magical Child be in charge. Allow her to pick out your outfit, choose what you'll eat, and decide who you'll spend time with.
- Schedule time for your creative work each week. Put that at the center of your life, rather than keeping it at the bottom of your list. Protect your creative time like a fierce mama bear. Block out one- to three-hour chunks to do whatever you love most: writing, cooking, painting, gardening, dancing, singing, playing an instrument, sewing, scrapbooking, and so forth. These don't need to be things that will earn you a living (although they can be). They are things that help you to feel more alive, passionate, and on fire. They're rooted in those activities from childhood that you most enjoyed.

Step into the Creative Tao

When the Magical Child completes the formation of our daemons, the Tao, also translated as "the Way," springs forth. This concept stems from an ancient Chinese manual on the art of living called the Tao Te Ching (pronounced "daw deh jing" and translated as the "Book of the Way"), by Lao Tzu, a contemporary of Confucius who lived around 500 BCE. We can also see the Tao as "the Middle Way." It's what flows forth from a fully integrated mandorla. When we hold the tension of the opposites within ourselves without resisting or turning away, a sacred river — or the Tao — flows through us. When we experience this flow, the doors to our creative potential open and lifetimes of healing and insight can transpire in a single moment. This is the space of miracles that simply cannot be explained with the mind but only understood with the heart. In these moments, everything seems right and in perfect divine order — no matter how messy the journey has been. Through this portal, works of creative genius and spontaneous healing are born.

Although we all yearn to fully step into this flow of grace, in fact most of us spend our entire lives avoiding it. As we've discussed throughout the book, we make the mistake of thinking that facing head-on what we most fear will destroy us, when, actually, it's the only thing that can truly save us. When we allow ourselves to stand in the chaos of life, with our hearts open and our minds relaxing into uncertainty long enough for the paradox of death and rebirth to reconcile, we experience the creative Tao, the Way.

The Tao is powerful. It builds worlds and it destroys them. It's entirely up to you to direct its currents. You are far mightier, my dear, than you give yourself credit for! Get clear on what you want to build and what you want to let go of. For example, if you're leaving a relationship or a job, don't hesitate. Trust your decision. End it and move on. Let the path before you open up as you take your next steps.

Don't wait to do this, because if we don't create, we die. We're not taught about the enormity of our creative potential as women, and nearly *every* woman I know is creatively blocked in some way. This isn't our fault. We're living in a time when art isn't valued, but if we don't embrace the innate artists that we *all* are, our demons win. If we don't embrace our true nature as creators, we cannot actualize lasting health or happiness. Don't let yourself become so busy that you forgo your real passions.

Our bodies scream loud and clear when we're not participating in the juicy, life-affirming, creative currents that they need to thrive. When I've neglected creative pursuits in the past, I've gotten depressed and tired. Some women develop autoimmune diseases. And don't think for another moment that you aren't creative. We are *all* artists. Creativity is the foundation of our existence and the means through which the divine manifests itself in the material world.

Let's live our way into the Tao. To live creatively is to eat life up, exactly as it is. Just because the world wants us to focus only on external pursuits doesn't mean we have to. We must devote time each day to our creative pursuits to bridge the divide between the lives we're living on the surface and the unlived ones within us. Take small steps to achieve this every day, allowing each one to serve and express your deepest Self.

The Heroine's Journey calls us back home to the unlived life within us. The creative impulse is the divine impulse when we use it toward a positive end and run it with intention. It's yours alone to define, and it need not be expressed in big, bold, or unusual ways. You don't need to be famous to be creative. Just create. Sprinkle fresh blueberries on your oatmeal or add a feather to your hat. Send postcards to friends and leave love notes for your sweetie. Creative energy can never, ever be depleted. The more you access it, the more you have.

Through your SHE Cycles, cultivate your creativity like farmers care for their crops. Plant new ideas in the spring, nurture them in the summer, harvest and then prune them in the fall, and leave your inner fields fallow in the winter. Your creative cycles help the world to heal and evolve. Together, let's learn to see our roles as mothers in more than just the biological sense. Let's merge with the Divine Mother in the Tao, giving birth to babies of all sorts.

Write the Vision for Your New Life

Ten years ago I attended a silent meditation retreat on the outskirts of Chiang Mai, Thailand, with one of my heroines. Buddhist teacher Tenzin

Palmo is the author of *A Cave in the Snow* and one of the first Westerners to be ordained as a Buddhist nun. As the title of her book suggests, she lived in a cave in northern India's Himalayas for twelve years, the last three of which were in strict, secluded retreat.

Sitting before us with serene stoicism, she told us about dreaming that she was locked in a prison. When she realized that her cell was unlocked, she burst out of it, ran down the hallways, and unlocked the doors to the cells of all of the other inmates. Much to her surprise, the others refused to leave their cells. Despite her pleas urging them to escape, they didn't budge. They wanted to stay in their rooms, enwrapped in the comfort of the familiar. Tenzin Palmo warned us that we all live in prisons of our own makings. Even though the door can open to freedom, that doesn't mean we'll all have the courage to claim it.

Now that we've dismantled the prisons of our own suffering through the processes laid out in this book, it's time to trade them for the unfamiliar territory of our new lives. We must remember that insight without action is useless. It's time now to leave the old and embrace the new. We've cultivated the skills for working with what is. Now it's time to partner with the potential for what could be. You have within and around you all the help and support you need to live your vision. Take the reins. Fully author your life. Don't *try*, just *become*.

And remember two things:

1. This is lifelong learning.
2. In creating the masterpieces of our lives, we're not escaping reality or trying to change it in any way.

As you move forward, don't expect the chaos, darkness, or pain to go away. That's not the point — far from it. Think back to chapter 4, when we discussed the two ways of working with life: actuality (being with what is) and potentiality (actively imagining what could be). As you create your life, make sure it involves relinquishing the need to seek pleasure or push away pain. Create your life in a way that truly *honors* life. The goal is not to be perfect, but to lead a sustainable and satisfying life in which you can be more fully yourself.

The Navajo call this paradigm "the Beauty Way," for everything we experience in life can be transformed into something exquisite. This view is a choice. Your mind *is* the mind of the Goddess, and your thoughts therefore hold the power to create reality. You're *that* powerful. During this visioning and your living of it, remember that in each moment you *choose* how to respond to and frame every experience. Your outer world will always offer you valuable feedback, reflecting to you your inner state.

Wherever you are right now, ready or not, just get started. Without delay, rise up to meet your life. The only way to do it wrong is to not do it. Align with your beautiful future that *wants* you to partner with it. Be deeply purposeful and intentional, attending to every little detail. Make it just the way *you* want it.

As you go, rest with the knowing that it's okay to proceed at your own pace — always. The external world often makes us feel such a sense of urgency, leaving us anxious, fearful of lagging behind, and overwhelmed. From that state, we're cut off from our inner resources. Instead, find and embrace the rhythm that allows *you* to thrive. The consequences of *not* doing this simply aren't worth it. Don't let anyone or anything rush you.

Include in your vision a daily practice and time for seasonal and yearly retreats. These allow you to keep training yourself to be with yourself as you are while affording you the space to digest the events of your life, learn your lessons fully, and dream new dreams. Be compassionate with yourself, and know that it may take time (some say *at least* sixty days) before you notice the big changes that come from transforming your old patterns. Stay with it, even if you can't see the results yet. Don't do it for someone else to love you more. Do it even if no one else notices. Empowerment comes from aligning your attention and actions with your SHE's truth, day after day. Build your new vision in concentric circles from your heart, fueled *by* your heart.

Dream a New Dream

To do this exercise, take two to three hours to yourself. It's best to do this after a yoga and meditation practice so you're coming from a deeply embodied, present place. Make it a sacred affair. Light some candles, pour some tea, take out your journal. Connect with your belly and your creative organs. Breathe into your heart. Activate the parts of your body needed to create your dream life *from within*.

- Write down, in the first person and present tense (e.g., "I feel," "I am"), your vision of how you would like your life to be if you could have it *exactly* as you wanted it. If you could be, do, or have everything you wanted, what would that ideal life look like? What are your greatest fantasies and creative ideas? What would make you incredibly happy? How would you live if you trusted yourself and expressed your unbridled power, fully? Be as specific as possible. Include all areas of your life (health, self-esteem, spirituality, support structures, relationships, family, finances, self-care, personal growth/education, creative expression, lifestyle, material possessions, leisure, adventures, contribution).
- Write down all the reasons why you don't think you can have what you want. Ventilate the limiting beliefs that are keeping you trapped inside the prison of your own making. When you see them all written down, ask your SHE to remove these beliefs and open up new pathways for receiving the abundance of your true nature.
- Ask yourself: Who will I be when this dream comes true?
- What's the song that only you can sing?
- What message does your SHE have for how to get from where you are now to that vision? Listen for Her answer and write it down.
- When you're finished, read your vision aloud and record it. Visit the vision often — in both its written and verbal forms. Read it before bed; listen to it during savasana after your yoga practice. If it's helpful, create a collage that represents this vision in colors, pictures, and symbols. Don't just *think* about it (that's fantasizing, not visioning). Each time you visit your vision, *feel it* in your body as if it's already here. Physically *love* it, as a prayer for your future self from your heart.
- Remember this equation for bringing your dream to life:

Manifestation = Clear Intention + Aligned Action

- Carefully choose the crops you want to plant, and then water those seeds daily.

Clarify Your Vision

Here are some ways to go even deeper with your new life vision:

- Create a "Life Vision" binder to store all of your goals and dreams. Keep this in your sacred space and return to it often.
- Curate an inventory of practices that will support you going forward. Look back over the practices shared in this book and others that you currently engage in (or want to engage in). Make a list of these resources to draw on, and put it in your binder.
- Clarify your top three goals for the next year. Make sure that they are steps toward the castle of your ideal life vision. Then identify three goals for each season, month, week, and day that will support those larger yearly goals.
- Schedule times to review, revamp, and revise at the end of each day, week, month, season, and year.
- What kind of inner and outer support do you need to actualize these goals? How will you get what you want? Consider teachers, mentors, therapists, courses, retreats, friends, spiritual family and community, free time, your rhythms/rituals/schedule, daily spiritual and self-care practices.
- What nourishes you? Consider people, activities, pets, foods, practices, movies, music, books, and so forth.
- Make a list of the patterns of self-sabotage that could get in the way of you fully living your new vision.
- What are some fears that come up for you about the idea of living your vision? Write them all down.
- What is currently preventing you from getting what you want?
- Who do you need to forgive? What messes do you need to clean up? What steps do you need to take in order to no longer hold anything against anyone for any reason?
- How do you define success? How will you know when you're successful?

- What are you ready to *stop* doing? Where are you settling for mediocrity through crazy busyness? What are you currently doing that doesn't feel like "you"? Where are you playing the victim or rigidly demanding your way?
- How do you want to define your womanhood going forward? Your sexuality? Divinity? Your work/public persona?
- What small risk will you take today to face your fear? Choose micro-behavioral "stretches" each day to help you become the woman who lives this vision. Stretch out of your comfort zone, daily, to morph new patterns into your nervous system.
- Continue to cocreate with your SHE every day during your practice by prayerfully asking for what you need and then looking for synchronistic signs (in people and mundane, daily circumstances) to give you what you need.
- Say thank you. Graciously accept what is given to you. Continue to witness and partake in the everyday acts of Her grace all around you.
- Exercise your faith more and relax your doubt. Faith is trusting in the unseen more than in the seen. When you doubt the possibility of your vision manifesting, you block Her grace from making it so.

Consult with Your Inner Family about Your New Vision

Once you've painted the picture of your new life, it's time to change your inner beliefs to support it. Remember, if you don't transform your negative patterns, you'll pass them on to others until someone steps up to the plate to clear the family karma. As the sovereign, loving parent, call all of the members of your inner family together. Exercise your strong and flexible ego as the leader of your inner home. Share your vision with your inner family. Take the time to hear everyone's fears, requests, and feedback. Take each inner self seriously, receiving all input with acceptance and graciousness, because you can only actualize your vision through harnessing the help of *all* aspects of your psyche. Even just one rebellious straggler can sabotage your dreams.

Your Inner Family Meeting

Here's a visualization for holding this inner family meeting, inspired by my energy alchemist mentor Hiro Boga.[1]

To listen to this guided visualization, go to www.TheBookofSHE.com /practices, to download the audio file. I've also included it in written form here.

Have your journal and a writing utensil nearby and come into a comfortable seated or lying position. Remember: this is rich, deep material. Work at your own pace. Be gentle with yourself. Pause the audio at any point if you feel like you need more time. If you start to feel overwhelmed, come back to your breath and the process of getting grounded.

Close your eyes and follow your attention down the golden thread of your midline into your belly center. Feel the rise and fall of your breath in your belly. Take ten slow, deep, and even breaths. With each one, inhale clarity and awareness and exhale tension and tiredness. After those ten breaths, establish your grounding cord and stay with it until you feel a steady flow of earth energy in your body.

Now take a breath over the front surface of your heart. Feel your heart and palpate its center. Prepare a sacred space in your heart for a family ritual with all of your inner selves. What does this place look like? Is it a chapel or a serene place in nature like a forest or beach? Make sure it's a safe and secluded space with a clear boundary. If you're indoors, the boundary can be walls, and if you're outside, it can be a circle of stones, a grove of trees, or a horseshoe-shaped beach. In the center of the circle see a communal seat in the form of a mother's lap that's big, warm, and unconditionally loving.

Call a circle of your inner selves into your heart. Gather your inner family with the intention of not leaving anyone out of your life plan. Once everyone is gathered, ask them to make themselves comfortable and tell them why they're here. Tell them that you invited them because they are important members of your inner family and you want their support and involvement in birthing a new vision for your life. Explain to them, in as much detail as possible, what's going on in your life right now. Tell them what you're in the midst of and what you're desiring to create. Paint for them the picture of your ideal life. You can pause this audio anytime and give yourself more space with this process.

Invite all your inner selves to have their turn to come and sit on the mother's lap to speak their truths. Safe from criticism and judgment, they can speak honestly, ask for what they need, and share their wisdom. Ask them how they feel about these changes. What are their thoughts and feelings about them? One or more of them might have wisdom or insights to share that you hadn't before considered. Ask them what they need to feel safe and supported as you move toward this vision together. Also ask them to support you in this new life. You need one another and the gifts you all hold in order to create this. Remember that your inner selves might not agree with one another. See beyond their fear, anger, and anxiety. You don't need them to agree with one another and you don't need to agree with them, but everyone *does* need to feel safe and honored in order to live peacefully together.

As you listen to them, write down anything you hear. Notice what each self looks like. What are their names? How old are they? What is your interaction like with them? Write down what it's like for you to stay open, receptive, and respectful as you hear them out. Call forth each self's inner wisdom and unique expression of love. Invite each of your inner selves to show you its heart, for it holds the very essence of this inner self. Remember that even your more challenging parts have valuable things to share and gifts to offer too.

There might be certain inner selves that have felt challenged for a long time. They might need extra time and support to decompress when they come onto the lap in order to change a long-standing pattern. In certain cases, you might need to call a negotiator or an ally, such as your Divine Masculine or Inner Crone, to help with one of these conversations. Remind each of your family members that it's not a forgotten fragment, but it's part of your sacred whole.

When all of your inner selves have spoken and you feel complete, thank each one of them. Make a date to meet with them again to give them an update on your creations and to see how they're doing. Let each self know that it belongs here, every step of the way. When every part

of you supports and contributes to the life you're shaping, your life becomes richer and much easier. Everything that you do becomes more
coherent and joyful because you don't feel like you are being pulled in
a million different directions. When these inner selves start to feel more
harmonious, your presence itself becomes a blessing to the world. When
your inner home is at peace, you can accomplish a lot of beautiful and
powerful things in your life.

To conclude, see each of your inner family members leaving the circle. See your sacred space dissolving in your heart. Place your right hand
on your heart and your left hand on your belly. Take a few deep breaths.
With eyes closed, feel the physical space that you're in from your heart.
And when you're ready, slowly open your eyes.

After you've written down everyone's responses in your journal, come
back to your center. From your sovereign SHE, determine the next steps
to take as the leader and advocate for your entire inner family. Ask yourself:

1. What do *I* really, truly want here?
2. What is the best thing for *me* to do in this situation, regardless of
   what other people think?
3. What would I do if it really didn't matter to anyone else?
4. How can what I truly want also take into account all of the concerns
   I just heard from my family of inner selves? Where is the compromise here?
5. What concrete actions can I now take, based upon all this information that I've just gathered?
6. How does it feel in my body? (When you feel a big YES from within,
   you know the process is complete. If not, there are still some inner
   voices that need dialoguing with.)

Celebrate Your Accomplishments

Do you hear that? It's the quiet hum of completion. *Hmmmm*...Pat yourself on the back, sister — you have *every* reason to feel *really* good about

any and *everything* you've accomplished on this journey, and in your life at large. Drink in this moment. Feel it as a complete accomplishment, knowing that, right now, you don't have to do *anything* else. It's time to gather around the fire you've built and feel nourished by its warmth. Rest here a while, by the hearth of your success, rather than being a self-help junkie, frittering on in search of the next big fixer-upper in your life. Let right here, right now be enough. Allow this experience — and any big life undertaking — to gestate for at least nine months before taking on something new. Through this, you will remember to always create space to enjoy the life you've worked so hard to create.

Learn the art of celebrating your life as it is, because celebration generates *more* celebration. Plan something special for yourself. What will that be? Pause and receive the huge amount of grace that you're sitting in, and feel how victorious you already are — *right now*. Rest in the comfort of a job well done, releasing any guilt you might carry about that. Know that it may take a while for this journey to fully integrate. Be patient. Practice faith and trust by resting in this pause, waiting and opening. Allow for the seeds planted deep within you to sprout in their own time. Also, don't berate yourself if you feel like you should have taken this journey years ago. Trust how divine timing operates in your life. You're exactly where you're supposed to be. You're right on time.

Since paradox is always at play, at another level recognize that on the Heroine's Journey of your life there is no "there," no finish line, no resting place. We're constantly evolving. Transition never ends! As Zen teacher and author Natalie Goldberg instructs, "Sometimes we fail for a week, a month, a year, a decade. And then we come back, circle the fire. Our lives are not linear. We get lost, then we get found. Patience is important, and a large tolerance for our mistakes. We don't become anything overnight."[2]

Relinquish the belief that your deepest wounds will ever fully heal. Most likely they won't. They'll keep getting triggered throughout your life as you travel the narrowing spiral toward your death. As you now know, these wounds aren't your enemy; they're the keepers of your daemons, holding your impetus to evolve. Knowing this, abandon the assumption that you can ever live completely free of obstacles.

Take the seat in the center of your life by getting out and living your life. I mean, *really* live. Don't be afraid to, at times, ditch your to-do list, turn off your computer, and put your phone away for a bit. Paint your life in bright colors and be sure to let it be multidimensional, bridging inner and outer, seen and unseen. Make your whole life your masterpiece, using your body as your paintbrush. Keep putting aside how you want things to be and *just act*. Remember: in your joy you heal the world, and your way *is* always the Way. Don't be afraid of your power, take responsibility for the gifts you have been given, and never, ever take them for granted.

Protect your gifts fiercely, for within them resides your Divine Child of Love. To magnify your gifts, be more generous with them. Always be on the lookout for ways to uplift another person, because we all know how life can be a hell realm at times. Reach out and do whatever you can, whenever you can, to ease another's suffering. Being the lone Heroine is not the end of the road, for there's only so far that we can journey on our own. At a certain point, we have to learn to partner, serve, and celebrate one another.

Feel immense devotion, respect, and gratitude for those who have aided you on your journey, in any way. Always revere anyone who has ever given you anything valuable. Spiritual teachings are the greatest wealth in this world, and we live in a time when we've forgotten that. Regard your teachers in the highest light. Simultaneously, take them off their pedestals, accept their full humanity, and give them permission to make mistakes, just like you. Then live and pay forward whatever they've taught you to the best of your ability. As you heal and awaken to greater and greater levels of joy, love, and wholeness, it's your turn to serve.

Closing Ritual:
The Blessing and Appreciation Circle

Let's gather to conclude our journey. Feel all the women who have taken the Heroine's Journey and all the men who have undergone the Hero's Journey — past, present, and future — joining together now in a sacred circle. Feel the dignity of *your* seat in this configuration of gods and goddesses. No one can take this seat from you, and no one can give it to you. It's yours alone to claim. Remember that this seat *never* leaves you; it follows you wherever you go. Know that you can call upon this circle at any time in your life when you need support and remembrance of who you are and what you're most devoted to serving in this lifetime. This is your tribe of soul sisters and brothers. Remember that, here, anything is possible for your life. *Anything.*

Outside of this circle, envision all of your teachers, parents, guides, and ancestors in another circle around you (and their teachers in an even wider circle). From your heart, feel your gratitude radiating out toward them, landing in their hearts as a magnetic, indestructible bond between you and them. With one hand pressed to your heart, share any words of appreciation with your teachers and this community that feel right for you. When your sharing feels complete, see all members of these concentric circles melting into a single rainbow light that rains down upon us all, dissolving into you as an experience of oneness. Visualize all of your obstacles melting, and your most radiant qualities shining through.

Feel every step of this Heroine's Journey etched into your heart. You know the Way now, and you can call upon it any time you need it. It lives in you, as you, in your own unshakable SHE. Through the endless cycles of life and death that you will continue to face in large and small degrees, remember that you are a Heroine, and no one or nothing can change that.

Welcome, my dear Heroine. From this point on you are already, always, and forevermore *home.*

The Dedication of Merit

To formally close our journey, let's follow the Buddhist practice of dedicating the merit of our actions for the benefit of all beings. Remember that "all beings" includes you, so as you recite these words, either aloud or silently, feel yourself absorbing the fruits of your inner work, while also extending them outward in all directions to nourish sentient beings everywhere. If it feels comfortable, place both hands together in a prayer position in front of your heart as you recite the following verses.

May all beings be happy,
May all beings be at peace,
May all beings be free from inner and outer danger,
May all beings be free of suffering, and the roots of
    suffering.

I dedicate the merit of my practice to all beings.
Namaste! And so it is! Amen! Ah ho! Yes, Ma!

Part V

The Homecoming

If you travel far enough,
one day you will recognize yourself
coming down the road to meet you.
And you will say
YES.

— Marion Woodman, *Coming Home to Myself*

Princess Tara

*Perhaps all the dragons in our lives are really princesses
who are waiting to see us act, just once, with beauty and courage.*

— Rainer Maria Rilke, *Letters to a Young Poet*

Boulder, Colorado; May 31, 2014

She's called by many names: Star, She Who Ferries Across, She Who
Saves, and the Mother of Mercy and Compassion. The Buddhist goddess
Tara, with her dedication to ceaselessly serving the liberation of all beings,
decided that there were too few women who had attained Buddhahood.
So she vowed, "I have developed *bodhicitta* ["awakened heart-mind" or
"mind of enlightenment"] as a woman. For all my lifetimes along the path
I vow to be born as a woman, and in my final lifetime when I attain Bud-
dhahood, then too I will be a woman."

Green Tara is a female Buddha of enlightened activity who embodies
compassion in action. This youthful, eternally sixteen-year-old goddess is
most often depicted sitting on her lotus throne with her right foot tucked
in toward her in mediation and her left foot stepping out into the world in
protection of sentient beings everywhere. Upon hearing the cries of the

world, she knows that to best serve, she needs to stay rooted in herself in order to alleviate the suffering of the masses. In this way, Green Tara reminds us that life as a Heroine is a continuous flow of giving and receiving. She models how to be fully in the world, and also beyond it — at home in both idealism and realism.

The final stage in our development is to become seamless, without boundaries, so that we can pass from outer to inner, inner to outer, without a break or disruption. At this point, we stop hiding behind the mask of our personas to protect our innermost selves, and, like Tara, we can finally be of true service to the world.

As I prepared to finish the rough draft of this manuscript, I signed up for a solitary retreat at Lama Tsultrim's Tara Mandala, a retreat center and temple for the Sacred Feminine, and to Tara in particular. Before I departed, I met with Sofia for guidance.

At the close of our session, Sofia advised me to cultivate a relationship with Green Tara while I was there, to help me complete this book. Her words of wisdom apply to all of us.

> The secret of Tara is that she's a princess. She's not a queen. She holds vulnerability, innocence, and the aliveness of the Goddess that women forever have complete access to. But you *have* to nourish it. You do this through combining yourself with things that are fresh, and applying your body to inhaling and exhaling the qualities that you revere in Her. You tussle with this until you realize that *you* are the power that you have recognized in Her.[1]

Chapter 13

Becoming a Whole
and Holy Heroine

There were no empty places in her soul,
no corners left untouched by love, not a shadow in her heart.

— Ken Wilber, *Grace and Grit*

"If you think you're enlightened," spiritual teacher Ram Dass warns, "go spend a week with your family."[1] Let's be honest: returning home may be the hardest part of any journey.

After I graduated from college, I lived in Thailand for nine years. While I was there, I promised myself that I would eventually go home to my birth land, my family of origin, and the wounds within my soul that those places triggered. Only when we go home do we see how far we've come and how far we still have to go.

However, in many ways it was harder for me to move back to the United States than it had been to uproot myself to go to Thailand in the first place. After any big journey, integration is a *very* challenging — but necessary and worthwhile — *process*.

Like everything else in life, our homecoming is a transition. It's not an arrival in a perfected reality. It's not about suddenly having all the answers and feeling forever safe and secure. No. The same ground rules apply for the homecoming as for the journey. There is no ground, there is no home, there is no safety, other than what we create within our own loving presence in this, and every, moment. This moment, right here, like this, is home. You, right here, like this, is home. *There is nothing else.*

We must come home with an increased willingness to relax into the questions and to trust and appreciate the mystery of this collective journey. We come home not to be superior but to be truly helpful and humble. We come home not to prove ourselves but to share who we truly are. We come home not to proclaim our truth from the rooftops but to express our own authentic voice, rooted in an indestructible inner conviction. We come home to be reminded of where we still need to grow and to soften our hearts even further into the suffering — our own and others' — that will never end.

We come home because, at last, we have found home within ourselves. We have found a wellspring of inner nourishment and ground that no one or nothing can ever take away. We come home not to be forever confident but to be able to continue to hold space for ourselves, and others, throughout the continued cycles of existence — especially death and the dark spells of fear, ignorance, and not knowing.

We come home in the spirit of generosity, sharing the bounty of our inner spheres with those around us (regardless of whether others are receptive to or appreciative of them). We come home to the place from which we were born, the place from which we began. Even though everything and everyone around us may be exactly the same as they were when we left, we know that we have irrevocably changed. We have lived lifetimes. We have died and been reborn thousands of times. We have loved and we have lost. We have found our true family — within us and in our own chosen communities. We have wept alone beneath the stars, and we have fallen asleep in our beloved's arms. When we go home, everything *looks* the same, but, in reality, *everything* is different on the other side of this journey — especially you. You are no longer a girl, nor are you just a woman. Now you are a Heroine. Not just any Heroine, but a whole and holy Heroine. The Heroine of *your own life.*

Before I leave you to live your homecoming, let's return to the woman who led us into our journey at the start of this book — Mary Magdalene.

While I did not know then why She visited me that Devil's Night, now the significance of Her presence rings clear.

Our Heroine, Mary Magdalene

As I reached the denouement of this book, and my own heroine's homecoming, I wondered if there was a feminine archetype that embodied our *entire* journey — one who begins as an ordinary human woman and, through the transformation of her suffering and Awakening, becomes a goddess. With this query, I recognized that this woman, this goddess, *is* Mary Magdalene. The entrance to this book and now the exit to it, She's the one who most fully expresses the full-spectrum humanity *and* divinity of the Heroine's Journey.

Both an ordinary woman and a timeless feminine archetype, Mary Magdalene is also known as the "apostle to the apostles," Jesus's beloved, a fully realized woman, and, as a result, a spiritual teacher and master in Her own right. She learned how to embody the wisdom teachings of Jesus, was the only one with enough devotion to witness His resurrection, and went on to walk the talk of Jesus's teachings while living *in* the world, not above it. She learned how to love in a way that cast out fear in Herself and others. She extends this holy love as Her greatest offering, even here and now. In a world devoid of female role models who fully exemplify the fruits of the Heroine's Journey, Mary Magdalene is the one who shows us what a woman who has done her inner work looks like. Even more, She's gone all the way, beyond gender distinctions to full spiritual realization.[2] For these reasons, Mary Magdalene is the best representation we have of a whole *and* holy heroine — a woman living for and as her SHE.

This is why Mary Magdalene is rising up from the collective unconscious, returning in droves to women — and men — around the world in dreams, visions, life crises, and books like this. Regardless of one's religious persuasions, the archetype of Mary Magdalene represents our fullest feminine potential. She reminds us to reach higher and further, toward all that we're truly capable of. Her return calls us to activate *all* aspects of ourselves, as one integrated, embodied, and forever free and loving SHE.

The Feminine Face of God

Like Mary, when we persevere on this path of feminine spiritual practice, following it all the way to the end, we too have the chance to arrive at our ultimate destination — full spiritual liberation.

In claiming our essential nature, we merge with Her source — the primal matrix that has held us all from the beginning. Here, we transcend gender and personhood to claim our Absolute nature, which has been called the Eternal Feminine, Sophia, the Feminine Face of God, and the Divine Mother. In Tibetan Buddhism, our essential nature is also known as Prajna Paramita, or the Primordial Mother of all the Buddhas. Although depicted in female form, her identity transcends all gender. She represents the enlightened quality of transcendent wisdom, insight, and the perfection of clear comprehension. The awakened heart-mind of supreme wisdom, Prajna Paramita is the highest potential that human beings can attain, the apex of our Heroine's Journey — beyond words and completely free from the limitation of concepts.

With insight into Prajna Paramita, we realize that the one serving, the one being served, and the compassionate action of service are all the same totality — there is no separate, continuous self to be found in any of these. This unifying, nondual, alchemical feminine is our *true* homecoming, on the Absolute level. These are not separate things, nor are they "things" at all. They aren't archetypes, deities to be worshiped, or states to attain or strive for. *They are who we truly are.*

This realization of the Feminine Face of God *is* the ultimate homecoming, residing within us all along, waiting to be actualized.

The Divine Mother's Blessing

If you're reading these words right now, you're one of the pioneering women who look out onto the vast landscape of a very uncertain future. The world needs something new from us, but we don't yet fully know what that is. We don't know exactly how or where we'll be called to act, but we all know — loud and clear — that we *are* being called. We're needed, and we need to get ready. We're in this together, united on a single front to perfume the world with the sweet rose scent of feminine wisdom once more.

Listen to Her. She is trying so very hard to get our attention. I need Her. You need Her. This world needs Her. We all must celebrate, remember, cry, and sing out to the Mother — in ourselves and in all things, because whatever you bless blesses you ten-thousand-fold in return. As a daughter of the earth, stand upon Her with dignity and reverence. Feel Her pulse as yours. Feel Her nourishment as ours. When we remember to open to Her as we all did so naturally as little girls, we allow the inexhaustible sweetness and mercy of the Divine Mother to bless our every act of kindness, giving us the renewed capacity to *always* hold what's here.

It's now time for *you* to live the journey that is *yours* to claim. Remember, whatever remains unhealed within you will haunt you until you face it. And whatever remains unhealed within you is, ultimately, only radically *good*. It's Her love calling you home. She's right there with you, every step of the way.

Sometimes when I lived in Thailand I'd come back to the United States for visits. Then whenever I'd return to Chiang Mai, I'd always find a note from my mom tucked away into a tennis shoe or a pant pocket: "Godspeed," she'd write. "I'm always right here with you, in your pocket. XO Mom."

We're forever in this together — mothers, grandmothers, sisters, and daughters. We love you so much. We believe in you. And you always have us in your back pocket too.

Acknowledgments

I had so many helpers during this journey that I don't know where to start! First, thank you to my beloved, Kogen Ananda Keith Martin-Smith. We met the day after my journey began — after my first visitation from Mary Magdalene — and I don't consider that a coincidence at all! You've been with me through every twist and turn, high and low. I truly couldn't have made it through this Heroine's Journey without your love and support. Only when I learned that I couldn't do everything on my own did my journey really begin. I love you so much. Thank you also to our sweet doggie daughter, Amia, who often sat at my feet (snoring) while I wrote these pages and hiked up Mt. Sanitas with me at the end of each long day of writing.

Thank you to my teacher, Sofia Diaz, for all the text messages, phone calls, practices, and meetings, each filled with fierce love and immense feminine wisdom. I treasure who you are and what you bring to this world. I love you and I bow deeply to you, in all your humanity and Sophia nature.

Thank you to my mom, Sara Sr., for your invaluable support and generosity — always.

I extend much gratitude to the healers and mentors who helped support my body, mind, and soul at various stages along the way: Sarah

Powers, Hiro Boga, Andrea J. Lee, Susan Aposyan, Dr. Nita Desai, Maggie Staedler, and Tracey Holderman.

Many thanks to my peer readers who offered invaluable comments: Peach Friedman, Tracey Blier, and Keith Martin-Smith. Also a great web of colleagues and friends helped me at various stages along the way: my editor, Georgia Hughes, for trusting this idea before it had any shape or form and for working with me as obstacles arose; excellent freelance editors; Tona Pearce Myers, for interior design and typesetting; Tracy Cunningham, for the beautiful cover art; Kim Corbin, for all your help with the publicity; and the entire New World Library team.

Much appreciation to Emma Teitel and Bari Tessler, for encouragement along the way; Chelsea Brady, for the Heroine's Journey diagram; Watz Base, for the steadfast virtual assistance to me and our community; plus Michael Greene and Janet Goldstein, for your legal help in the early stages.

I bow to my many unseen guides: my SHE, Mother Mary, Mary Magdalene, Archangel Michael, Green Tara, Dakinis far and wide, Machig Labdrön, the Buddha, Pippi Longstocking, Emily Dickinson, Marion Woodman, John Welwood, Carl Jung, Joseph Campbell, and so many others.

Thank you to all the pioneers in women's empowerment and spirituality on whose shoulders I stand, as well as to Maureen Murdock, for laying the groundwork with the Heroine's Journey; and to the Tara Mandala Retreat Center and Lama Tsultrim Allione, its founder and spiritual director, for an inspiring space to write.

I thank all the women who are part of The Way of the Happy Woman® community, especially the certified teachers, for your devotion and willingness to stand in the fire of your own transformation. It's such a privilege to work with you, and you inspire me every day to keep growing and serving.

Last, to all the men and women who have undergone the Hero and Heroine's Journeys, I bow to each and every one of you. Namaste.

Notes

Introduction

1. Liza Mundy, "Women, Money and Power," *Time*, March 26, 2012, http://content.time.com/time/magazine/article/0,9171,2109140,00.html.
2. Hanna Rosin, "The End of Men," *The Atlantic*, July–August 2010, www.theatlantic.com/magazine/archive/2010/07/the-end-of-men/308135.

Chapter 1. Leaving Your "Normal" Life

1. Tina Fossella, "Human Nature, Buddha Nature: On Spiritual Bypassing, Relationship, and the Dharma — An Interview with John Welwood," *Tricycle*, Spring 2011.
2. Maureen Murdock, *The Heroine's Journey* (Boston: Shambhala, 1990), 2.
3. Sara Avant Stover, *The Way of the Happy Woman* (Novato, CA: New World Library, 2011).
4. Murdock, *The Heroine's Journey*.
5. Ibid., 38–39.
6. Ibid., 29–32.
7. Christiane Northrup, MD, *Mother-Daughter Wisdom* (New York: Bantam, 2005), 24.
8. Elizabeth Gilbert, *Eat, Pray, Love* (New York: Penguin, 2006), 10.

Chapter 2. Entering Your Inner House

1. Emma Young, "Gut Instincts: The Secrets of Your Second Brain," *New Scientist* 2895 (December 15, 2012), 38–42.
2. Adam Hadhazy, "Think Twice: How the Gut's 'Second Brain' Influences Mood and Well-Being," *Scientific American*, February 12, 2010, www .scientificamerican.com/article/gut-second-brain.
3. "Grounding," Wikipedia, accessed April 15, 2015, http://en.wikipedia.org /wiki/Grounding.
4. Jill Satterfield, www.vajrayoga.com; used with permission.
5. John Welwood, *Perfect Love, Imperfect Relationships* (Boston: Trumpeter, 2007), 29.

Chapter 3. Healing the Mother Wound

1. John Hunter Padel, "Freudianism: Later Developments," in *The Oxford Companion to the Mind*, ed. Richard L Gregory (Oxford: Oxford University Press, 1987), 273.
2. Louann Brizendine, MD, *The Female Brain* (New York: Broadway Books), 15.
3. Lauren B. Adamson and Janet E. Frick, "The Still Face: A History of a Shared Experimental Paradigm," *Infancy* 4, no. 4 (October 2003), 451–73.
4. The University of Adelaide, "Can 'Love Hormone' Protect Against Addiction?" March 20, 2014, www.adelaide.edu.au/news/news69442.html.
5. Mark Epstein, *The Trauma of Everyday Life* (New York: Penguin, 2013), 18.

Chapter 4. Crafting a SHE-Centered Life

1. Shunryu Suzuki, *Zen Mind, Beginner's Mind* (Boston: Shambhala, 2011), 147.
2. Marion Woodman, *The Crown of Age* (Boulder: Sounds True, 2004).

Chapter 5. Dancing with the Dark Goddess

1. Marion Woodman, *Emily Dickinson and the Demon Lover* (Boulder: Sounds True, 2009).
2. Clark Strand, "Bring On the Dark: Why We Need the Winter Solstice," *New York Times*, December 19, 2014, www.nytimes.com/2014/12/20 /opinion/why-we-need-the-winter-solstice.html.
3. Thomas M. Heffrom, "Insomnia Awareness Day Facts and Stats," *Sleep*

Education, March 10, 2014, www.sleepeducation.com/news/2014/03/10/insomnia-awareness-day-facts-and-stats.

4. Woodman, *Emily Dickinson and the Demon Lover*.

5. Ken Wilber, *Grace and Grit* (Boston: Shambhala, 2001), 58.

6. Ibid., 58.

7. See www.sarahpowers.com.

8. Marion Woodman, *Conscious Femininity* (Toronto: Inner City Books, 1993), 28.

9. Sera Beak, *Red Hot and Holy* (Boulder: Sounds True, 2013), 119.

10. John Welwood shared this teaching at a retreat I attended with him in 2013.

11. Marion Woodman, *Holding the Tension of the Opposites* (Boulder: Sounds True, 2007).

12. Dalai Lama, *An Open Heart: Practicing Compassion in Everyday Life*, ed. Nicholas Vreeland (New York: Little, Brown, 2001; reprint, 2002), 21.

Chapter 6. Ending the War Within

1. Tony Dokoupil, "Is the Onslaught Making Us Crazy?" *Newsweek*, July 6, 2012, 24–30.

2. Tara Mohr, *Playing Big* (New York: Gotham, 2014), 3–5.

3. Brené Brown, *Daring Greatly* (New York: Gotham, 2012), 34.

Chapter 7. Unlocking the Magic in Your SHE Cycles

1. This information is from a handout I received several years ago from a workshop led by my friend Tracey Holderman (www.sourcemassage.com).

2. John Wijngaards, "Women Were Considered Ritually Unclean," accessed April 19, 2015, www.womenpriests.org/traditio/unclean.asp.

3. Brené Brown, *Daring Greatly* (New York: Gotham, 2012), 75.

4. Jim Loehr and Tony Schwartz, *The Power of Full Engagement* (New York: Free Press, 2003; reprint, 2005), 12.

5. Alisa Vitti explores a similar concept in her book *WomanCode* (San Francisco: HarperOne, 2014), 143–54.

6. Office on Women's Health, "(PMS) Fact Sheet," http://womenshealth.gov/publications/our-publications/fact-sheet/premenstrual-syndrome.html.

7. Harriet Lerner, PhD, *The Dance of Anger* (New York: HarperCollins, 2005), 1.

8. Ibid., 4.

Chapter 8. Meditating on Your Mortality

1. Tsoknyi Rinpoche, "The Four Thoughts That Change the Mind," www.tsoknyirinpoche.org/2575/web-teaching-i-2.
2. This translation is from teachings I've received from Sarah Powers, author and founder of Insight Yoga, www.sarahpowers.com.
3. National Institute on Aging, "Health and Aging: Menopause," January 22, 2015, www.nia.nih.gov/health/publication/menopause.
4. Christiane Northrup, MD, *The Wisdom of Menopause* (New York: Bantam, 2012), 69.
5. Ibid., 7.
6. Ibid., 30–32.
7. Marion Woodman, *Conscious Femininity: Interviews with Marion Woodman* (Toronto: Inner City Books, 1993), 88.
8. Crone definition from *The Oxford Pocket Dictionary of Current English,* 2009, www.encyclopedia.com/doc/1O999-crone.html.

The Golden Dakini

1. Tsultrim Allione, *Feeding Your Demons* (New York: Little, Brown, 2008), 14–15.
2. Ibid., 15.

Chapter 9. Unveiling the Sacred Heart of *Real* Feminine Power

1. Marion Woodman and Elinor J. Dickson, *Dancing in the Flames* (Boston: Shambhala, 1997), 50.
2. Tsultrim Allione, *The Mandala of the Enlightened Feminine* (Boulder: Sounds True, 2007).
3. Ibid.
4. Cynthia Bourgeault, *The Meaning of Mary Magdalene* (Boston: Shambhala, 2010).
5. Sera Beak, *Red Hot and Holy* (Boulder: Sounds True, 2013), 196–97.
6. Ibid., 197.
7. Bourgeault, *The Meaning of Mary Magdalene,* 59.
8. Pema Chödrön, *When Things Fall Apart* (Boston: Shambhala, 2000), 49.
9. This is a practice and perspective that I learned from Sofia Diaz, www.sofiayoga.com.
10. American Heart Association, "Facts about Heart Disease in Women," www.goredforwomen.org/home/about-heart-disease-in-women/facts-about-heart-disease.
11. "Heart," *Wikipedia,* accessed April 22, 2015, http://en.wikipedia.org/wiki/Heart.

Chapter 10. Turning On Your Brights

1. Tony Schwartz, "Overcoming Your Negativity Bias," *New York Times*, June 14, 2013, http://dealbook.nytimes.com/2013/06/14/overcoming-your-negativity-bias/?_r=0.
2. Brené Brown, *Daring Greatly* (New York: Gotham, 2012), 118.
3. Regena Thomashauer, *Mama Gena's School of Womanly Arts* (New York: Simon & Schuster, 2003), 59.
4. Clarissa Pinkola Estés, *Women Who Run with the Wolves* (New York: Ballantine, 1992), 1.
5. Ken Wilber, "Divine Pride and the Integral Movement," *Integral Life*, March 17, 2010, www.integrallife.com/video/divine-pride-and-integral-movement.

Chapter 11. Marrying the Divine Masculine

1. Sarah Powers, *Insight Yoga* (Boston: Shambhala, 2008), 11.
2. These reflections are from handouts I received at the Hoffman Process, www.hoffmaninstitute.org.
3. Tsultrim Allione, *The Mandala of the Enlightened Feminine* (Boulder: Sounds True, 2007).
4. Marion Woodman, *The Crown of Age* (Boulder: Sounds True, 2011).
5. Marion Woodman and Elinor J. Dickson, *Dancing in the Flames* (Boston: Shambhala, 1997), 135.
6. Mihaly Csikszentmihalyi, *Creativity: The Psychology of Discovery and Invention* (New York: HarperCollins; reprint, New York: Harper Perennial, 2013), 71.
7. Marion Woodman, *Conscious Femininity: Interviews with Marion Woodman* (Toronto: Inner City Books, 1993), 86.

Chapter 12. Birthing Your Beautiful Life

1. See www.hiroboga.com.
2. Natalie Goldberg, *The True Secret of Writing* (New York: Atria Books, 2014), 28.

Princess Tara

1. From a private session with Sofia Diaz (www.sofiayoga.com) on March 31, 2014.

Chapter 13. Becoming a Whole and Holy Heroine

1. Ram Dass, Facebook post, November 24, 2014, www.facebook.com /babaramdass/posts/861701467195253 (accessed June 25, 2015).

2. Cynthia Bourgeault, *The Meaning of Mary Magdalene* (Boston: Shambhala, 2010), 36.

Index

About the Author

Sara Avant Stover is leading a movement to inspire women to come home to their true selves. A yoga and meditation instructor, bestselling author, inspirational speaker, and founder of The Way of the Happy Woman®, Sara graduated Phi Beta Kappa and summa cum laude from Columbia University's all-women's Barnard College. After a cancer scare upon her graduation, she moved to Thailand and embarked on a decade-long healing odyssey throughout Asia. Since then, she has gone on to uplift tens of thousands of women worldwide. The creator of the world's first women's yoga teacher training, the SHE School, the SHE Retreat, and Reversing Our "Curse," Sara has been featured in *Yoga Journal*, the *Huffington Post*, *Newsweek*, and *Natural Health* and on ABC, NBC, and CBS. She lives in Boulder, Colorado, with her fiancé, Keith, and their dog, Amia.

Join The Way of the Happy Woman® Community

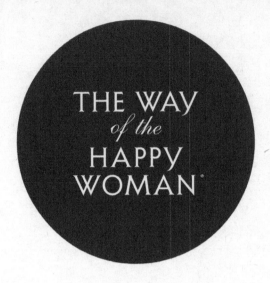

The Way of the Happy Woman invites every woman to join our gentle revolution by challenging the status quo and finding happiness within. We resuscitate and proliferate ancient feminine wisdom by providing women with safe and sacred spaces to come home to themselves and their true power — their vulnerability. When we first feel at home in ourselves, we can then feel at home *just as we are* in the world.

Connect with Our Global Community Online
(#WayOfHappyWoman, #SHE, and #BookofSHE)

Website: www.TheWayOfTheHappyWoman.com

Facebook: www.Facebook.com/WayOfHappyWoman

Twitter: www.Twitter.com/WayOfHappyWoman

Instagram: www.Instagram.com/TheWayOfTheHappyWoman.com

Pinterest: www.Pinterest.com/SaraAvantStover

The Book of SHE Free Practice Resources

For additional free support during your Heroine's Journey, you can download free audio practices, such as:

- Guided visualizations for Entering Your Inner House, Connecting to the Earth, Meeting Your SHE, Meeting the Dark Goddess, and holding a meeting with your inner family
- A full-color PDF map of the Heroine's Journey
- Access to our private SHE Circle on Facebook for sharing and connecting along the way

Receive these practices at www.TheBookofSHE.com/practices.

Interested in Joining One of Our Programs?

We offer in-person workshops, retreats, and teacher trainings worldwide, as well as online learning programs. Some of these include:

- **The SHE School:** An online group-mentoring immersion and spiritual-practice immersion (www.TheSHESchool.com)
- **The SHE Retreat:** Weeklong retreats in paradise (www.SHE retreat.com)
- **Reversing Our "Curse":** A homestudy e-course to help you unlock the magic in your SHE Cycles (www.ReversingOurCurse .com)
- **The Way of the Happy Woman Seasonal Retreats:** Yoga, meditation, and life-balance seasonal retreats with Sara or one of our certified teachers near you (find one via the link to the events schedule below)
- **Women's Yoga Teacher Training:** Learn how to teach yoga and meditation to women in all seasons of life (www.Womens YogaTeacherTraining.com)

View our entire schedule of events here:
www.TheWayoftheHappyWoman.com/calendar

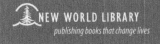